Dear Joe —

Thank you so much
for all your support

Carol Flannery

A Surgeon's Path

Kahyun Yoon-Flannery • Carla Fisher
Marc Neff
Editors

A Surgeon's Path

What to Expect After a General Surgery Residency

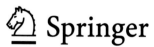 Springer

Editors
Kahyun Yoon-Flannery
Sidney Kimmel Cancer Center
Jefferson Health New Jersey
Sewell
NJ, USA

Carla Fisher
Department of Surgery
Indiana University School of Medicine
Indianapolis
IN, USA

Marc Neff
Center for Surgical Weight Loss
Jefferson Health New Jersey
Cherry Hill
NJ, USA

ISBN 978-3-319-78845-6   ISBN 978-3-319-78846-3   (eBook)
https://doi.org/10.1007/978-3-319-78846-3

Library of Congress Control Number: 2018948707

Printed on acid-free paper

This Springer imprint is published by the registered company Springer International Publishing AG part of Springer Nature
The registered company address is: Gewerbestrasse 11, 6330 Cham, Switzerland

To our children, Jamie, Andrew, and Dylan,
To Ella, Leo, Max, and Nathaniel,
and to all the hardworking surgical
residents.

Preface

June 2016 was my 15-year anniversary of graduating from my surgical residency. June 2001 was the time I felt like I was leaving the protective nest of being a resident and had to enter the real world. I felt bittersweet nostalgia. I felt on top of the world as a chief resident. I knew how to get anything done in the hospital for my patients. I knew who people were, how to work the computer system, every shortcut, every door combination, and I had the respect of everyone around me. They had watched me grow from a hatchling intern afraid of his own shadow, fearing I would kill a patient by inserting a nasogastric tube, to the surgical chief who could do an appendectomy skin to skin before his attending made it in from home to scrub the case. Looking back, I didn't know what I didn't know.

I remember feeling nostalgic for those days when I didn't have so much uncertainty and worry in my life. A quick inventory included worry about malpractice lawsuits, timely completion of my patient charts on the latest and greatest electronic health record, would the proposed addition of the nursing practitioner for the bariatric surgery program budget be approved, how did my personal life disintegrate when all I was trying to do was work hard and take care of patients, and the list went on and on.

It was in that same month that a soon-to-graduate chief resident set fire to an idea inside of me that had been smoldering for quite some time. I was in the operating room, the case was done, the orders were being put into the computer, and I suggested to my chief some words of wisdom about what comes after graduation. She hungrily consumed every word lamenting all the things she hadn't learned in residency and some trepidation and fear about what comes next. I shared with her the idea of putting the collective wisdom of years of mistakes we surgical attendings make in a tome and providing it to residents at graduation. She suggested that the current chief residents could even contribute based on their experiences their final year as they prepare for graduation/fellowship/new jobs. I offered maybe even some help from other professionals in related and even dissimilar fields. The idea caught fire. We started to solicit authors, asking if they would be willing to contribute. An idea was pitched to a publishing company. It was accepted. Spreadsheets were created. Commitments were obtained. The fire grew to an inferno.

Herein contains the collective wisdom of what happens after residency, by so many who had to learn wisdom only by making mistakes. The goal, however, should be to learn before the mistake is ever made. Or at least to recognize the mistake for what it is, and then maybe the mistake won't be so devastating or so much of a setback. I don't believe in blindly approaching the maze of life, but by intelligently approaching it. You don't have to have it figured all out to enter the maze, but you don't have to hit every dead end either.

Not everyone can be a surgeon. Being a surgeon takes commitment, discipline, curiosity, and patience. This book is meant for those who have already made it to being a surgeon, but they now need a "quick reference map," a pathway for what comes next, so they minimize their chances to get lost.

Today's surgeon has to be part technician, part IT specialist, an administrator, a clinician leader, and likely half a dozen other roles I haven't mentioned. The chapters are meant to be little nuggets of helpful wisdom in those roles. Like appetizers. Helpful information in a condensed format. Easy to read. Suggestions offered. Lessons provided. Some chapters are similar in content, as there may be different lessons to learn from the same challenge depending on your age, gender, or point in your career.

We hope this will aid you in your quest to become an attending surgeon: the person we all looked up to as an early medical student, in complete control in and out of the operating room, fully confident, without uncertainty or fear.

Cherry Hill, NJ, USA   Marc Neff

Acknowledgments

This book has been a long project in the making. The sheer volume and number of chapters included in the book certainly would not have been possible to compile together without the participation of each individual contributing author from all over our country. I am grateful for their participation, their words of wisdom, and also for their patience over multiple emails from myself for their drafts. Without them, this book would not have been possible.

This book certainly would not have been possible without the guidance and leadership from our senior editor, Dr. Marc Neff. Not only was this book his original idea for many years, he was involved in every aspect of the development of the book. Without his guidance, the book nor I would be where we are now.

Secondly, I would like to thank my Fellowship Program Director, advisor, mentor, and hustler sister, Dr. Carla Fisher, for eagerly agreeing to come onboard on the project and pushing me along the way. Her keen and unusual sense of honesty and attention to detail have improved this book in so many countless ways, and for that and for many other things, I am forever grateful.

Lastly, I would like to dedicate this book to my dear husband, companion in life, biggest supporter, baby daddy, and partner, Peter M. Flannery, Esq. He has seen through it all, from graduate school, commuting into the city for a research position, medical school, a brutal surgical residency to a challenging surgical fellowship and finally in first practice. Without his support, I would not be where I am in my career, nor would I have had the courage to continue my demanding surgical career all the while not compromising our ambition for a large family. My hope is that every single medical student, surgical resident, and young surgical attending reading this book will hopefully understand that despite the difficult days and years that have accompanied us along the way, all of it can and will be possible if you have the will for it, especially if you have a supportive partner standing beside you. I know I did and I am eternally grateful.

January 2, 2018

Kahyun Yoon-Flannery

Contents

Part I Surgical Fellowships

1 Fellowship Applications 3
Linda Dultz and Elliott R. Haut

2 Fellowship Interviews 7
Mary T. O'Donnell and Lucy M. De La Cruz

3 Trauma and Surgical Critical Care Fellowship 11
Jonathan Nguyen and Asanthi M. Ratnasekera

4 Breast Surgical Oncology Fellowship 19
Rose E. Mustafa and Kahyun Yoon-Flannery

5 Burn Fellowship 25
Neha Amin

6 Colon and Rectal Surgery Fellowship 29
Mary T. O'Donnell and Nicole M. Saur

7 Complex General Surgical Oncology Fellowship 35
Shanel B. Bhagwandin and Devin C. Flaherty

8 Vascular Surgery Fellowship 41
Holly Graves

9 Minimally Invasive Surgery Fellowship 45
Roshin Thomas and Stefanie Haynes

10 Plastic Surgery Fellowship 49
Sarah N. Bishop and Nakul Rao

11 Transplant Fellowship 55
David P. St. Michel

Part II   How to Find a Job

12   Where to Look for a Job After Residency   63
Jonathan Nguyen and Thomas J. Cartolano

13   Job Applications   67
Rose E. Mustafa and Jonathan Nguyen

14   Interviewing for Your First Job   71
Asanthi M. Ratnasekera

15   Contract Negotiation   75
Kahyun Yoon-Flannery and Jonathan Nguyen

16   Gender Inequality in Compensation in Medicine and Surgery   81
Kahyun Yoon-Flannery

17   Applying for Privileges and Licensure   87
Jonathan Nguyen

18   Moving   91
Anuradha Reema Kar and Elliott R. Haut

19   Malpractice Pearls for the Young Surgeon   97
Kunal T. Vani and Matthew J. Finnegan

20   Academic Medicine   101
Jonathan Nguyen and Bryan C. Morse

21   Hospital Employment   105
Thomas J. Cartolano

22   Lessons Learned in Private Practice   109
David M. Schaffzin

Part III   After Finding a Job

23   Partners   115
Marc Neff

24   Medical Economics   117
Alan M. Neff

25   Gifts   123
Marc Neff

26   Marketing   125
Steven M. Pandelidis

27   Finding a Mentor   129
Marc Neff

28 **Setting Up Your Office** 131
    John D. Paletta

29 **Building a Program** 141
    Adair De Berry-Carlisle and Marc Neff

30 **Lawsuits** 145
    Marc Neff

Part IV After Starting Your First Job

31 **Preparing for Your First Day on the Job** 153
    Linda Szczurek

32 **Dealing with Your Clinic** 157
    Linda Szczurek and Nicole M. Saur

33 **Navigating Electronic Medical Records** 163
    Robert Neff and Jonathan Nguyen

34 **First Call with Your First Emergent Case as an Attending** 169
    Linda Szczurek and Holly Graves

35 **How to Avoid Disasters in the Operating Room** 171
    Louis Balsama

36 **When to Ask for Help** 179
    Linda Szczurek

37 **Finding the Balance of Letting Residents Operate While Managing
    Patient Safety** 181
    Linda Szczurek

38 **Choosing the Right Staff** 185
    Robert Neff and Marc Neff

39 **How to Be Smart with Case Selection** 195
    Gustavo Lopes

40 **Building Your Practice** 199
    John D. Paletta

41 **When Your Patient Dies** 205
    Marc Neff

42 **Innovation** 207
    John R. Bookwalter

43 **Future Technology in Healthcare** 209
    Robert Neff

44 Interacting with Residents 213
Sandra R. DiBrito and Elliott R. Haut

45 Professionalism 221
Linda Szczurek

46 Research 227
Fabian M. Johnston and Elliott R. Haut

47 Continuing Medical Education/Maintenance of Certification 235
Carla Fisher

48 Board Exams 239
Marc Neff

**49 Becoming a Fellow of the American College of Surgeons
and American College of Osteopathic Surgeons** 241
Asanthi M. Ratnasekera and Marc Neff

Part V Long-term Goals and Planning

50 Learning New Procedures 245
Marc Neff

51 Robotic Surgery 247
Matias J. Nauts and Roy L. Sandau

52 Military Surgery 251
Gustavo Lopes

53 Five-Year and Ten-Year Plans 255
Marc Neff

54 Changing Practices 257
David M. Schaffzin

55 Leadership Development 263
Paula Ferrada

Part VI Maintaining Your Health

56 Work-Life Balance 271
Daniel Neff

57 Stress Management 275
Daniel Neff

58 Burnout 279
Marc Neff

59 Diet and the Surgeon 281
Marc Neff

60 When Is It a Good Time to Have a Baby? 283
Kahyun Yoon-Flannery

61 Social Media and Your Professional Presence Online 287
Christian Jones and Elliott R. Haut

62 Mindfulness 291
William D. Stembridge

63 Divorce 297
Marc Neff

64 Life as a Surgeon from a Spouse's Perspective 299
James J. Cavello, Peter M. Flannery, and Melissa Cartolano

Index 303

Contributors

Editors

Kahyun Yoon-Flannery, DO, MPH Sidney Kimmel Cancer Center, Jefferson Health New Jersey, Sewell, NJ, USA

Carla Fisher, MD Department of Surgery, Indiana University School of Medicine, Indianapolis, IN, USA

Marc Neff, MD, FACS, FASMBS Center for Surgical Weight Loss, Jefferson Health New Jersey, Cherry Hill, NJ, USA

Authors

Neha Amin, DO Rowan University School of Osteopathic Medicine, Stratford, NJ, USA

Louis Balsama, DO, FACS General Surgery Residency Program, General and Bariatric Surgery, Rowan University School of Osteopathic Medicine, Stratford, NJ, USA

Shanel B. Bhagwandin, DO, MPH Division of Surgical Oncology, Department of Surgery, The Icahn School of Medicine at Mount Sinai, New York, NY, USA

Surgical Oncology and Hepatopancreatobiliary Surgery, Jupiter Medical Center/ Jupiter Medical Specialists, Jupiter, FL, USA

Sarah N. Bishop, MD Division of Plastic and Reconstructive Surgery, Mayo Clinic, Rochester, MN, USA

John R. Bookwalter, MD, FACS Brattleboro Memorial Hospital, Brattleboro, VT, USA

Melissa Cartolano, MSN Frankfurt, IL, USA

Thomas J. Cartolano, DO Trauma Surgery and Surgical Critical Care, Advocate Christ Medical Center, Oak Lawn, IL, USA

University of Illinois, Chicago, IL, USA

James J. Cavello, MBA Johnson & Johnson, Horsham, PA, USA

Adair De Berry-Carlisle, DO, FACOS, FACS Trauma and Acute Care Surgery, Surgical Critical Care, St. David's South Austin Medical Center, Austin, TX, USA

Lucy M. De La Cruz, MD Division of Endocrine and Oncologic Surgery, University of Pennsylvania, Philadelphia, PA, USA

Sandra R. DiBrito, MD Department of General Surgery, Johns Hopkins University School of Medicine, Baltimore, MD, USA

Linda Dultz, MD, MPH Division of Burn, Trauma and Critical Care, Department of Surgery, University of Texas Southwestern Medical Center, Dallas, TX, USA

Paula Ferrada, MD, FACS Director of the Surgical Critical Care Fellowship, Surgical and Trauma ICU, Virginia Commonwealth University, Richmond, VA, USA

Associate Professor of Surgery, Virginia Commonwealth University, Chicago, IL, USA

Matthew J. Finnegan, MD, FACS General Surgery, Lourdes Medical Associates, Haddon Heights, NJ, USA

Carla Fisher, MD Department of Surgery, Indiana University School of Medicine, Indianapolis, IN, USA

Devin C. Flaherty, DO, PhD, FACOS Valley Health Surgical Oncology, Winchester, VA, USA

Peter M. Flannery, Esq Bisgaier Hoff, Haddonfield, NJ, USA

Holly Graves, MD Jefferson Health New Jersey, Voorhees, NJ, USA

Elliott R. Haut, MD, PhD, FACS Division of Trauma Surgery and Critical Care, Department of Surgery, Johns Hopkins University School of Medicine, Baltimore, MD, USA

Stefanie Haynes, DO Philadelphia College of Osteopathic Medicine, Philadelphia, PA, USA

Fabian M. Johnston, MD, MHS Department of Surgery, The Johns Hopkins University School of Medicine, Baltimore, MD, USA

Christian Jones, MD, MS, FACS Division of Acute Care Surgery, Department of Surgery, Johns Hopkins University School of Medicine, Baltimore, MD, USA

Anuradha Reema Kar, MD Acute Care Surgery, Trauma, Burns and Critical Care, Department of Surgery, Johns Hopkins University School of Medicine, Baltimore, MD, USA

Gustavo Lopes, DO General, Laparoscopic, and Robotic Surgery, Chairman Department of Surgery, Martin Health System, Stuart, FL, USA

Bryan C. Morse, MD Trauma/Surgical Critical Care, Department of Surgery, Grady Memorial Hospital, Emory University School of Medicine, Atlanta, GA, USA

Rose E. Mustafa, MD Breast Surgery, Saint Peter's Breast Center, New Brunswick, NJ, USA

Matias J. Nauts, DO Laparoscopic and Robotic General Surgery, Christus Surgical Group Lake Charles, Lake Charles, LA, USA

Alan M. Neff, MBA, HCM Neuro Diagnostic Devices, Prescott, AZ, USA

Daniel Neff, MD Department of Psychiatry and Human Behavior, Sidney Kimmel Medical College, Thomas Jefferson University, Philadelphia, PA, USA

Marc Neff, MD, FACS, FASMBS Center for Surgical Weight Loss, Jefferson Health New Jersey, Cherry Hill, NJ, USA

Robert Neff, BSc Digital Innovation and Consumer Experience Group (DICE), Thomas Jefferson University and Jefferson Health, Philadelphia, PA, USA

Jonathan Nguyen, DO Division of Trauma and Critical Care, Department of Surgery, Morehouse School of Medicine, Atlanta, GA, USA

Mary T. O'Donnell, MD Department of Colon and Rectal Surgery, Department of Surgery, Ft. Belvoir Army Hospital, Arlington, VA, USA

Assistant Professor of Surgery, Uniformed Services University, Bethesda, MD, USA

John D. Paletta, MD, FACS The Georgia Institute for Plastic Surgery, Savannah, GA, USA

Steven M. Pandelidis, MD WellSpan Surgical Oncology, York, PA, USA

Nakul Rao, MD Department of Surgery, Drexel University College of Medicine, Philadelphia, PA, USA

Asanthi M. Ratnasekera, DO Crozer-Keystone Health System, Upland, PA, USA

Roy L. Sandau, DO, FACOS Department of Surgery, Jefferson Health New Jersey, Cherry Hill, NJ, USA

Nicole M. Saur, MD Division of Colon and Rectal Surgery, Department of Surgery, University of Pennsylvania, Philadelphia, PA, USA

David M. Schaffzin, MD, FACS, FASCRS Drexel University College of Medicine, Philadelphia, PA, USA

St. Mary Medical Center, Center for Colon and Rectal Health, Inc., Langhorne, PA, USA

David P. St. Michel, DO, MPH Division of Transplant Surgery, University of Maryland School of Medicine, Baltimore, MD, USA

William D. Stembridge, DO Advanced GI Minimally Invasive and Bariatric Surgery, Anne Arundel Medical Center, Annapolis, MD, USA

Linda Szczurek, DO, FACOS Jefferson Health New Jersey, Cherry Hill, NJ, USA

Roshin Thomas, DO Rowan University School of Osteopathic Medicine, Stratford, NJ, USA

Kunal T. Vani, DO General Surgery, Rowan University School of Osteopathic Medicine, Stratford, NJ, USA

Kahyun Yoon-Flannery, DO, MPH Sidney Kimmel Cancer Center, Jefferson Health New Jersey, Sewell, NJ, USA

Part I
Surgical Fellowships

Chapter 1
Fellowship Applications

Linda Dultz and Elliott R. Haut

Introduction

So you've made it almost to the end of your general surgery residency, congratulations!!!! The fellowship interview process is about to begin for the vast majority of residents reading this book. Overall, the process is similar to applying to surgery residency, except the number of people interviewing for the same fellowship spots is much smaller. It is very likely you will see the same people on the interview trail, and these same people will become your colleagues for decades to come. So, as always, be professional and courteous throughout the entire process.

Application Documents

Start the process early!!! It doesn't matter what fellowship; they all require similar documents. Begin your research by knowing your deadlines. Most fellowship programs now participate in the National Resident Matching Program (NRMP). This website is critical to review prior to applying for fellowship. Use it to identify which fellowships and programs participate in your match and what the deadlines are (i.e., submitting applications and rank lists) and to review match data from prior years. Give yourself, your program director, and all your letter writers plenty of time to

L. Dultz, MD, MPH (✉)
Division of Burn, Trauma and Critical Care, Department of Surgery,
University of Texas Southwestern Medical Center, Dallas, TX, USA
e-mail: Linda.dultz@utsouthwestern.edu

E. R. Haut, MD, PhD, FACS
Division of Trauma Surgery and Critical Care, Department of Surgery, Johns Hopkins
University School of Medicine, Baltimore, MD, USA
e-mail: ehaut1@jhmi.edu

© Springer International Publishing AG, part of Springer Nature 2018
K. Yoon-Flannery et al. (eds.), *A Surgeon's Path*,
https://doi.org/10.1007/978-3-319-78846-3_1

Table 1.1 Commonly required documents for fellowship applications

Letters of recommendation (three letters, one from program director or chair)
USMLE Scores
ABSITE Scores
Medical school transcript
Medical school diploma
Curriculum vitae
Personal statement
State Medical Licensure, Drug Enforcement Agency (DEA) registration

compile the materials needed for your application. Request these items about 6 months in advance in order to give your letter writers and registrar offices ample time to gather these documents. A list of documents we recommend you obtain in advance are listed in Table 1.1.

Mentoring

One of the most crucial points to emphasize in this chapter is the importance of a good mentor (or, ideally, a mentoring team). Mentors can make or break your career depending on what they can or cannot offer you. Here are some key points when choosing a mentor:

1. Choose someone well known and respected in your chosen field. While it is easiest to find someone in the department where you are training, it must be stressed that this person does not need to be part of your department. A well-respected sponsor can successfully advocate for you when applying for fellowship. While there is often some overlap, there is a distinct difference between sponsorship and mentorship.
2. Select an academic/research mentor who is well published and can mentor you through various academic projects. Whether these are book chapters, papers, or presentations, a good mentor will teach you the academic side of surgery and stress how to do this well. Most mentors will be well established in their field and will already have project ideas for their mentees to work on. If you will be pursuing an academic career, use these opportunities to learn about grant writing, statistics, and writing papers, things that this type of mentor should be extremely proficient in.
3. A good mentor should also care about your personal growth outside of the operating room. They should help you find balance between your personal and professional life. Someone who cares about your career more than his or her own is the definition of a great mentor. They should help you get where you want to, not force you to go where they want you to be.

Networking

If you're fortunate enough to know well in advance what field you are going to specialize in, then make sure to network as much as possible. Fellowship programs are small, and many program directors know each other. They will also likely know most of the candidates prior to interviewing based on past interactions at conferences—use this to your advantage. Many candidates will do research in their area of interest and will present at various meetings throughout their residency years. Ask your mentors and sponsors to introduce you to their peers and let you tag along to invitation only events. Take every opportunity to meet as many people in the field as possible. Even if that person is not where you want to go for fellowship, you never know where your first job will be or who will move to another department. Maintain these relationships throughout the year via email and social media.

Letters of Recommendation

There are a few key points to discuss prior to requesting these documents.

1. Very carefully select the people to write your letters. Don't automatically choose only the division chief at your program.
2. Have an updated copy of your CV ready to give your letter writers when requesting a letter of recommendation. They may know how great you are on clinical rotations, but not realize all the other great things you have done which make you an excellent overall candidate.
3. Choose people well known in the field you are applying to and people that have worked closely with you.
4. Have a letter of recommendation from either your program director or chair. Use it if required, but don't feel compelled to if it is not required and you feel other letter writers will promote you better.
5. Request these documents well in advance.

Scheduling Interviews

The majority of fellowship applicants will still be in their general surgery residency during the interview process. Preparing for interview season as far in advance as possible will help you immensely. Try to request lighter rotations during this time frame. Doing this will make it easier to take time off to travel during interview season. For example, it's probably a bad idea to rotate on your chairman's service and schedule ten interviews for pediatric surgery in the same month. Being on a rotation with lighter hours, fewer inpatients, and less call makes it is easier to find coverage while you are away. Put some favors in the bank ahead of time (i.e., extra weekend or holiday calls), so when you ask, your fellow residents will more likely say yes. Check with your program leadership (program director, coordinator, administrative chief) to get the specifics on how much time you can miss and when it can occur.

Interviews

Unlike medical school and residency, where your paper application (i.e., test scores, publications) weighs heavily on where you are accepted, many fellowship interviews are more heavily based on your character. Fellowship directors realize that if you have gotten this far, most likely you are clinically and technically sound in and out of the operating room. Therefore, fellowship interviews are often meant to find a good "fit" between an applicant and a program. It is important to realize that while programs are interviewing you, you also have to critically interview the program.

We recommend practicing the interview process with a mentor or colleague prior to starting interview season. There are several resources out there that give examples of common questions asked on the interview trail. Examples of organizations that provide questions that are asked and questions to ask include the American College of Surgeons (ACS) and the Association of American Medical Colleges (AAMC). Review these resources in order to help you prepare some answers and create a list of questions ahead of time.

Choosing a Program

Similar to choosing a residency program, your personal and professional goals should align with the program you end up at. Making a list of your top priorities before starting the interview process is important, as this may limit your search early on. If being at a high-end academic center is important, this will eliminate many programs prior to interviewing. Geography is important to almost all applicants, and this will eliminate programs on location alone. To some geography may mean a specific part of the country. To others, it means being in any big city or somewhere with warm weather. How close do you want to be to your family? Does your spouse need a job? Are you willing to spend a year (or 2) in different cities? Whatever your priorities are, list them clearly, and know them before you begin the application process. This planning will keep you organized and focused during interviews and help narrow down which programs meet your goals.

During the interview process, ask where prior fellows have been hired after finishing fellowship. If you want to do academics, pick programs that have a history of placing graduates at the universities you might want to work at later in your career. This gives you an idea of what jobs will be available to you and how the faculty mentors fellows during their job search.

Remember that the match is a binding agreement. Don't list any program you are not willing to attend.

Chapter 2
Fellowship Interviews

Mary T. O'Donnell and Lucy M. De La Cruz

Introduction

You're in! If you have been offered an interview at a fellowship program, that means you have something the program liked, and therefore you have a good chance of matching with that program. Now don't blow it! No really, the interview is an opportunity for both you and the program to determine if it is the best fit for you. It is important to match to the program best for you, but it is also an opportunity to choose mentors, the type of practice you want to work in for a year or 2, and where you will be happy. The interviewers are similarly looking for someone who will be happy at their program and will become part of their community. Furthermore, programs are usually looking for candidates who are driven by similar interests, whether this is in research, type of practice, innovation, or teaching among other qualities.

The fellowship application process can be expensive. After spending ~$500 for 30 applications, you will still have to fund your travel, accommodations, and incidentals while attending fellowship interviews. Flights plus hotel can set you back $500 for an interview on the same coast, and traveling across country can be $750–$1000. Set aside $7000–$15,000 for a longer interview season. Social media can provide a means for coordinating with other interviewees to share rental cars or even hotels/accommodations depending on your level of comfort with other interviewees. We would recommend creating an excel spreadsheet to keep track of expenses because you can write these off on your taxes the following year.

M. T. O'Donnell, MD (✉)
Department of Colon and Rectal Surgery, Department of Surgery,
Ft. Belvoir Army Hospital, Arlington, VA, USA

Assistant Professor of Surgery, Uniformed Services University, Bethesda, MD, USA

L. M. De La Cruz, MD
Division of Endocrine and Oncologic Surgery, University of Pennsylvania,
Philadelphia, PA, USA

© Springer International Publishing AG, part of Springer Nature 2018
K. Yoon-Flannery et al. (eds.), *A Surgeon's Path*,
https://doi.org/10.1007/978-3-319-78846-3_2

Your fellowship interview is your opportunity to demonstrate the professional and mature surgeon you have become over the last 5–7 years, as well as your desires and interests for your future career. The following chapter is designed to provide advice for you to give the best representation of yourself and help you determine which programs have what you are looking for.

Show Respect and Deference for Those Interviewing You

Do your research! Read the biographies of the people you are interviewing with and look at what their research interests are and where they trained. It is possible that they trained at the same institution as you and they may know your current attendings and mentors. Your research or activities may be an area of interest that they share.

Be on time (e.g., 5–10 min early). I remember distinctly being 10 min early to an interview and was one of the last interviewees to show up.

Make sure the night before you see how far the interview location is from where you are staying and plan accordingly.

Be grateful; thank your interviewers for the opportunity to interview. If a program is one of your top choices, a short "thank you" email a few days to a week after the interview solidifies your interest. An actual handwritten thank you note to the program director is classy move to separate yourself from other applicants at a competitive program but is not always necessary.

First Impressions Are Everything!

Look professional—Wear a freshly pressed suit, no lint or awkward wrinkles. First impressions can contribute to a number of interviewer judgments about interviewees. You have 10–15 min for these highly intelligent and successful people to determine if they want to train you. Don't let the first 30 seconds interfere with that. Impress them.

Gentlemen—Wear a professional suit and a tie. Shave or keep your beard well kept. Similarly, have your hair looking kempt. You should look professional, and the interviewers should be able to focus on your credentials and not be distracted by your appearance.

Ladies—Wear a professional suit or a dress. Wear appropriate but sensible and comfortable shoes—they are often taking you on tours and you may be walking quite a distance that day! Just like the men, your goal in appearance is to look professional, not distracting.

Body language is important. Maintain good posture and make eye contact with all interviewers. Smile. Be upbeat. How you look is how you feel. Even angry surgeons do not want to work with someone who is unhappy at their fellowship interview!

Be Prepared to Discuss Anything in Your Application

Before you go into the interview, review your application. Be prepared to talk about anything you say in the application, because all of it, especially the personal statement and hobbies, is fair game.

You will be questioned about your education, honors or awards, and research experience and publications. Yes, *Even* that poster presentation you did as a medical student about 10 years ago can be a point of discussion, especially if the person you are interviewing with has an interest in this field so pay particular attention to connections with your application. If there is a medical mission or unusual hobby that you put on your CV—make sure you review it. You don't want to sound like you don't have a clue about the experience because they will think you lied on your CV. That is an absolute *Red flag*. This seems difficult to believe, but these interviews can actually be 10 months after you submitted the application and you may forget your most recent additions.

Make sure you have an idea of what you want to do and where you want to do it. In other words, be up front about your interest in academic versus private practice career or what your future career goals are.

So now, you have arrived at the interview. You are early, you look like a million bucks, and your heart rate is 120. Take a deep breath and remember that they asked you to come because they liked and respected your application. You academically deserve to be there. The interview is where you and the program determine whether or not you will be happy and succeed there. Now take another deep breath and relax…you are about to wow those in the interview.

First make sure to introduce yourself and call the attending by his/her name (i.e., Dr. Smith), and thank them for the opportunity to interview. Be prepared for up to 2–3 interviewers in one room. Be yourself. This advice seems like a cliché, but it is true. The interview is formal, but remember to keep a sense of humor. Channel your nervous energy into enthusiasm.

Don't be afraid to say, "I don't know" in reply to some questions. Some interviewers may push a particular line of questioning intending to find the point when you have to say, "I don't know."

Give short answers to the questions. Interviews usually last between 10 and 30 min, so time your responses accordingly. You don't want to spend too much time on any one question.

Don't be afraid to ask questions—plan ahead of time for two or three questions that are relevant to the program, i.e., Do you have dedicated research time? How much minimally invasive/robotic surgery do you do? Do we have moonlighting opportunity? It's important to ask questions that you can easily find answers for. For instance, if you already know that they have dedicated research time, perhaps you could ask what previous fellows have focused on during their research time.

Make sure you obtain email contact information. This includes the program director, the attendings who you interviewed with, the program coordinator, everyone! Follow-up emails are *Important*. Some programs will not give you their

email, but you can send them a postcard by snail mail. Whatever you have to do—
Follow up.

Make a list of all the programs you interview at and write down the pros and the cons. We recommend you do it as soon as you are done because you are likely to forget. At the end of the interview season, you can narrow it down to your top choices using the list you have made along the way.

Something no one ever mentions prior to the interview season is that it is important to socialize with your fellow applicants during interviews and interview season. Remember that they will be your future colleagues. We created a social media account for all the fellowship applicants the year we applied, and it is still maintained as a forum for questions for those subscribed to the account. Bottom line is these people will be your peers in the national society meetings and can be helpful partners in coordinating fellowship activities (especially if you are the only fellow at your program).

Suggested Reading

Gladwell M. Blink. The power of thinking without thinking. Boston: Little, Brown and Company; 2007.

Chapter 3
Trauma and Surgical Critical Care Fellowship

Jonathan Nguyen and Asanthi M. Ratnasekera

Introduction and History

The field of trauma surgery began as the Committee on Fractures by the American College of Surgeons in 1922 [1]. In the 1960s and 1970s, attention was drawn toward trauma after the publication of *Accidental Death and Disability: The Neglected Disease of Modern Society*. This publication highlighted the severity of accidental deaths in the USA and the need for more organized trauma systems [2, 3]. The need for more well-trained trauma surgeons was evident. However, the first formal trauma surgery fellowship was not developed until 1975 in the Maryland Institute for Emergency Medical Services. Since then it has seen several advances in number of fellowships as well as the focus.

To date, there is no accrediting board for *trauma surgery* or even *acute care surgery*. The ACGME and ACOS offer board certification for *surgical critical care*. The specialty is technically broken down into several arms: surgical critical care, trauma surgery, acute care surgery (ACS), and rescue surgery.

Surgical Critical Care

This specializes in education related to the management of critically ill trauma and surgical patients. The fellowship, and subsequently the career, focuses on how to manage critically ill patients suffering from sepsis from various intra-abdominal

J. Nguyen, DO (✉)
Division of Trauma and Critical Care, Department of Surgery, Morehouse School of Medicine, Atlanta, GA, USA
e-mail: jnguyen@msm.edu

A. M. Ratnasekera, DO
Crozer-Keystone Health System, Upland, PA, USA

© Springer International Publishing AG, part of Springer Nature 2018
K. Yoon-Flannery et al. (eds.), *A Surgeon's Path*,
https://doi.org/10.1007/978-3-319-78846-3_3

11

catastrophes, severely injured trauma patients, burns, and other surgical patients. A pure surgical critical care fellowship is typically 1 year in duration. Physicians from multiple fields such as anesthesiology and emergency medicine are able to participate in this fellowship.

Trauma Surgery

This part of the fellowship trains surgeons to triage and run resuscitations on the traumatically ill patient, coordinate and manage their care, perform research, and organize outreach for injury prevention. These fellowships can range from 1 to 2 years. The first year mostly is devoted to surgical critical care, and the second year may concentrate on a combination of acute care surgery and trauma service responsibilities.

Acute Care Surgery (ACS) or Emergency General Surgery

This relatively new fellowship grew from the realization that trauma surgeons are less frequently operating and more often coordinating the care of their injured patients with other services (orthopedic surgery, interventional radiology, neurosurgery, etc.). The American Association for the Surgery of Trauma (AAST) set forth guidelines that these 2-year fellowships should provide a broad experience in a wide range of surgical subspecialties. The intention was that graduates would be able to manage basic orthopedic and neurosurgical emergencies and have more experience in general surgery, trauma, emergency surgery, and surgical critical care. The initial implementation of these programs has yielded varying experiences from institution to institution, and further improvements are being made. That said, it is the growing trend that many programs are transforming to the acute care surgery (ACS) model. This fellowship is 2 years. Usually the first year is concentrated on 9–12 months of surgical critical care, while the second year is a rotating year among several services such as trauma, hepatobiliary, and cardiothoracic surgery. While it offers no specific certification, graduates are able to sit for their surgical critical care boards and able to get hands on experience on gaining knowledge and technical experience in a wide variety of organ systems. This should prepare the surgeon to learn how to gain rapid exposure during an austere case in a trauma patient.

Rescue Surgery

This aspect of the fellowship teaches the surgeon how to manage a complicated patient who may have had prior surgeries that have failed and need an expert for further management of the patient's disease process or surgical complications.

Unfortunately, in reality, this delineation of programs is not so clear. There are surgical critical care fellowships that offer a strong trauma component. They are afforded the trauma training experience, and 9 months of surgical critical care are required for the critical care boards. Other programs offer almost exclusively a critical care experience in which fellows rarely interact with the trauma team or operate. There are then 2-year surgical critical care fellowships. Though they are not technically ACS fellowships, they afford the extra year of surgical experience with some ability to modify the experience to the fellow's needs.

Which Program Should I Choose?

Selecting a program that suits your needs may at times be daunting. When making your selection about what path to follow, the critical question is what you as the applicant want and what you need to round out your training. Selecting a program that offers good education in critical care is of utmost importance to gain the knowledge and experience to pass the surgical critical care boards. The question that remains is whether your general surgery experience in residency has prepared you or not in order to pursue a 2-year acute care surgery combined fellowship. Two-year programs give you the extra time to hone your skills, solidify your decision-making pathways, and gain mentorship. One-year programs allow fellows who require extra time to refine their skills in trauma or for those who only want critical care.

You may also choose to complete a fellowship year to gain mentorship. This would be a great time to make connections with program directors and departmental chairs to further your surgical education. We have also used our fellowship years to advance our academic profile by being engaged in writing chapters for texts and research manuscripts and presenting at conferences such as Eastern Association for the Surgery of Trauma (EAST) and American Association for the Surgery of Trauma (AAST).

A 2-year program is not necessarily better than a 1-year program. Your selection should be directed toward filling gaps in your training and helping you obtain the job you want. Sources such as EAST and AAST offer websites that help categorize the programs (http://www.east.org/career-management/fellowships
http://www.aast.org/list-of-aast-approved-programs). These program websites can help shed light on what they have to offer. Often the best resource is to contact programs directly to ask questions about what the program involves.

Application and Interview Process

After extensive research you will be at the point of applying to select programs. The Surgical Critical Care Program Directors Society has created Surgical Critical Care and Acute Care Surgery Fellowship Application Service (SAFAS) (https://safas-sccpds.fluidreview.com/). The online website allows you to enter application information and select the programs that you would like to apply to. Usually SAFAS is open for applications in January of the year prior to your anticipated start of fellowship with a deadline in August. For example, if you are looking to start fellowship in August 2018, you will be applying in January–August 2017. During this time you will receive calls or emails for interviews. The application requires your CV and a personal statement. It also requires for you to have three letters of recommendation. At least one of those letters should ideally be from a trauma surgeon that you have worked with closely.

After submitting your application, it is important to introduce yourself to the program directors of the programs you are interested in and make them aware of your interest in their program. A simple email would be sufficient in this case. This would also be an opportunity for you to ask questions prior to your interview date.

During the months of May through September, you will be invited for multiple interviews depending on how many programs you have applied to. Usually, you will be invited to cocktails and a dinner event prior to the date of the interview. This is a great chance to meet the current fellows, faculty, and program director in a casual environment. Take this opportunity to be inquisitive, ask questions, and observe the relationships between the faculty members and fellows. Ask the fellows about their current call schedule, education opportunities, and opportunities for growth. Keep in mind, if you are interviewing for a 1-year fellowship, the current fellows may be brand new and may not have all the information you may ask. Make your hotel and travel arrangements and attempt to keep your interview dates organized. Make sure they don't interfere with other interview dates.

On the day of the interview, you are expected to be on time and dress in professional attire. Your interview may be an all-day or half day event. Either way come prepared. Make your travel arrangements to leave later in the evening so that you will not have to rush to leave an interview early. Pack lightly in case you have to check out of your hotel room before your interview time. You may have to bring your luggage with you to the interview.

Come prepared with questions to ask during your interview process. Study the faculty list and their background including where they trained and their areas of research. This will give you an idea of who could potentially help you advance your research and academic interest if you were to be accepted into the fellowship. During your interview, you may be given the opportunity to attend morning report. This is an excellent opportunity to observe the roles of the residents, fellows, and the attendings. The questions you should have in mind are: is morning report educational to the residents and fellows? Who presents the consults, admissions, and cases from the last 24 h? Is the discussion about these cases educational and advances the understanding of the patient disease process? After morning report you will have the opportunity to tour the facility, call rooms, and trauma bay. You will also have individual interviews with multiple faculty and the program director. Lunch may or may not be provided, either way you should be prepared with snacks and refreshments. During your interview, you will be asked what type of training you are looking for in a fellowship. It is important to realize what your gaps are in your current training and education and which areas you would like to improve during your fellowship.

After your interview, it is recommended that you reach out to the faculty and program directors that interviewed you and send them a "thank you" for the opportunity to be interviewed by their program.

Match Day

The National Resident Matching Program (NRMP) website allows you to rank your selection of programs. You may be familiar with this process from going through residency application process. The deadline for submitting your rank list is usually in September. The match day for Surgical Critical Care and Acute Care Surgery fellowships is usually in October. Congratulations if you have matched! If not, there is always an opportunity to "scramble" into programs. The website allows you to access the programs that did not match. You will have the opportunity to call these program directors for an opportunity for a phone interview and hopefully be offered a position in a fellowship.

The need for general surgeons who will perform emergency general surgery and care for trauma patients is on the rise. This need was met with the adoption of the acute care surgery model in many institutions. This need is also met by the demand for more fellowship-trained surgical intensivists and trauma surgeons. There has been an increase in the amount of applicants and fellowship spots through the years (Fig. 3.1).

This not only demonstrates the rising need for fellowship-trained trauma, surgical critical care, and acute care surgeons but also the increase in competition for these fellowships.

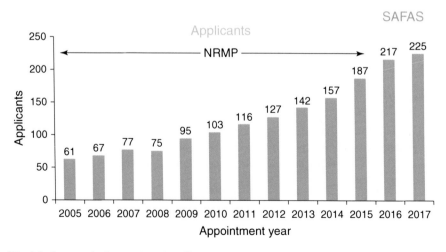

Fig. 3.1 Increase in the number of applicants and number of spots through the years (Data from SAFAS)

Fellowship Years

Graduation day from residency has just passed. You said your goodbyes to your attendings, staff, and co-residents that you have built relationships with for the past 5–7 years. Now you are on your first day at your brand new fellowship. You are learning your way around a large university hospital most likely with multiple fellows, co-fellows, and residents. You meet your faculty and staff for the first time. You are wondering what your day and responsibilities are going to be. So what are some important things to achieve for your fellowship years? As we mentioned earlier, for most your fellowship years are used to hone your decision-making skills and surgical technique and also develop mentorship. It is completely up to you and where you see your deficit may be. In our experience, we used these years to be educated in the principles of critical care, trauma resuscitation, and managing complicated surgical patients. We have also developed important relationships with the program directors and other faculty members who are successful in the field. This is of utmost importance to your career, as they may be able to help you publish your next big research manuscript, be invited to write a chapter for a textbook or even help you get a job when fellowship is done.

Once you start your fellowship, you must identify your role as a fellow. In many programs, the fellow is viewed as a junior attending and the responsibilities are as such. You are responsible for conducting rounds in the ICU; teaching residents, students, and other midlevel providers; and performing simple bedside procedures without supervision. The fellow is expected to take more of a leadership role as the year progresses.

The call schedule for fellows will vary depending on the institution. Taking call is an excellent opportunity to practice being a junior attending, making decisions by yourself but still having an experienced attending's input on your decision. This is also a great opportunity to teach residents and students who may be taking call with you, where you can walk a resident through a case and solidify your decisions by discussing the case and the rationale of your decision.

Key Points

- Trauma and surgical critical care fellowships come in different forms. It is up to you to decide which type of fellowship will suit your needs.
- Be prepared to ask questions during your interview and observe the faculty and fellows.
- The application process for surgical critical care is convenient with the advent of SAFAS.

- Matching to surgical critical care programs has become more competitive in the last several years due to an increase in demand for fellowship-trained surgeons and the rising applicant pool.
- Fellowship years are crucial to gain the knowledge and experience that was lacking from your prior training.

References

1. American College of Surgeons. Trauma. Available at: https://www.facs.org/quality%20programs/trauma. Accessed on 19th March 2017.
2. Reilly PM, et al. Training in trauma surgery: quantitative and qualitative aspects of a new paradigm for fellowship. Ann Surg. 2003;238:596–603. discussion 603–4.
3. National Academy of Sciences (US) and National Research Council (US) Committee on Trauma & National Academy of Sciences (US) and National Research Council (US) Committee on Shock. Accidental Death And Disability: The Neglected Disease Of Modern Society. Washington, DC: National Academies Press; 2014.

Chapter 4
Breast Surgical Oncology Fellowship

Rose E. Mustafa and Kahyun Yoon-Flannery

Application Process

Breast surgical oncology fellowship is generally a 1-year fellowship training available to candidates who have completed a general surgery or ob-gyn residency and who are board-eligible/certified surgeons. Some programs offer an optional second year of training focused on research. Applicants must apply through the Society of Surgical Oncology (SSO) (http://www.surgonc.org) Online Match System to participate in the match. As of the writing of this chapter, there are 46 SSO-approved training programs, which offer one to four fellowship positions per program each year.

SSO publishes instructions and a time line on their website each year. Candidates apply in the summer between their PGY fourth and fifth year. The SSO Online Match System Application usually closes mid-June. After candidates complete the application and submit the required documents on their Online Match System, SSO will send out reference letter requests. Interview offers will then be made via email from each program. SSO publishes a calendar of program-specific interview dates each match cycle online, and interviews generally extend from August through October. There are usually 2–3 programs per each interview date; therefore you may have to choose between different programs offering interviews. Each program usually offers two different interview dates to accommodate the applicants' schedules. If there is a program you are interested in and were not offered an interview initially, keep in mind that as some candidates must choose between programs, or interview

R. E. Mustafa, MD (✉)
Breast Surgery, Saint Peter's University Hospital,
Saint Peter's Breast Center, New Brunswick, NJ, USA

K. Yoon-Flannery, DO, MPH
Sidney Kimmel Cancer Center, Jefferson Health New Jersey, Sewell, NJ, USA

© Springer International Publishing AG, part of Springer Nature 2018
K. Yoon-Flannery et al. (eds.), *A Surgeon's Path*,
https://doi.org/10.1007/978-3-319-78846-3_4

dates don't coincide well, there may be some cancellations. Respectfully contacting programs later in the interview season for possible reconsideration of your application can be an option, although may not be received well by all institutions.

After interview season is complete, rank list will be due from both the programs and the applicants. After submitting the rank list, if you wish to withdraw officially from the match, you will have to contact fellowship@surgonc.org. Match Day is usually November 30. Results of the match will be announced individually via email. Historically SSO published the match result listed by each training program; however in recent years, this has no longer become widely available.

The key to having a successful match is to complete your application as early as possible, secure a good number of strong recommendation letters (three required, up to five accepted), and have a strong interview in person. Even prior to the Match System opening up, you should be gathering your application material, working on your personal statement, and revising your CV. Many successful candidates have their application files nearly completed by the time the system opens up.

The match rates for the past 6 years are listed in Table 4.1. Alarmingly, every year there are about 20–40% of unmatched candidates.

What else can an applicant do to boost their application, other than having perfect ABSITE scores, pages of first author publications, gleaming letters of recommendation as well as a riveting interview every time? One thing that had been encouraged to us was becoming a member of the SSO as well as the American Society of Breast Surgeons (https://www.breastsurgeons.org) (ASBrS) as soon as you are interested in breast surgery. It is not difficult to become *candidate* members of either organization as resident physicians, and this will also entitle you to lower registration fees for meetings and access to educational materials. It also demonstrates to individual programs that you indeed are interested in dedicating your life to the treatment of breast disease. These societies offer tremendous network and research opportunities, including but not limited to electronic access to the Annals of Surgical Oncology as well as multiple other online journals, continuing medical education programs, self-assessment programs, leadership opportunities, and volunteer opportunities. They both offer access to a career center to view current job listings.

Programs seek strong confident individuals who will uphold a high standard of training, ethics, practice, and ongoing research.

Table 4.1 Breast fellowship match statistics, courtesy of the Society of Surgical Oncology

Year	No. of applicants	No. of fellowship positions	Match rate (%)
2010	63	45	71.4
2011	63	43	68.3
2012	76	43	56.6
2013	69	54	78.2
2014	96	61	63.5
2015	88	62	70.5
2016	89	64	71.9

Fellowship Training

Comprehensive guidelines for training breast surgeons have been developed by the SSO to include the following main educational objectives: breast imaging, breast surgery, community service and outreach, genetics, medical oncology, pathology, and plastic and reconstructive surgery and rehabilitation. Under each heading, there are specific objectives that a fellow is required to meet during his/her fellowship training. While each fellowship program is required to offer a minimum of 2 months' training in surgery, the main goal of this fellowship training is to truly expose you to a multidisciplinary management of a patient with a breast complaint (Table 4.2).

ASBrS offers a "Fellows Program" containing multiple educational tools. In addition, there is a Web-based program called Breast Education Self-Assessment Program (BESAP) which includes a pretest and a posttest containing 59 questions that cover the categories as below:

- Advanced breast imaging
- Anesthesia/pain management
- Basic breast imaging
- Benign disease
- Cancer management
- Clinical trials
- Core measures
- Ethics, professionalism, medical/legal
- Medical oncology
- Oncoplastic surgery
- Surgery
- Breast cancer survivorship
- Palliative care
- Breast pathology
- Radiation therapy
- Risk assessment and genetics

Once you have completed the pretest, you receive an immediate score, and a score of 75% or higher is considered passing. Only then are you eligible to use the provided breast manual throughout your fellowship year. At the completion of your year, you are required to take the posttest.

Table 4.2 Sample breast fellowship schedule

Rotation	Duration (week)
Surgery	24
Medical oncology	4
Radiation oncology	4
Radiology	4
Pathology	2
Plastic and reconstructive surgery	2
Physical therapy	1

Table 4.3 Breast fellowship requirements by SSO

Procedure	Number required	Notes
Breast ultrasound		
Observation	30	
Hands on	15	
Percutaneous procedures	13	FNA, cyst aspiration, seroma aspirations, percutaneous needle sampling
Partial mastectomy or diagnostic excisional biopsy	50	Palpation guided, image guided, oncoplastic partial mastectomy
Mastectomy	40	Total mastectomy, skin-sparing, nipple-/areolar-sparing mastectomy
Axillary sentinel lymph node biopsy	50	
Axillary lymph node biopsy complete	5	Level 1, 2
Medical oncology	15 New breast cancer, recurrent 15 Follow-up visits	
Radiation oncology	15 New breast cancer consults 5 new breast cancer 15 Physics reviews or follow-up	
Pathology	8 Cancer case sign-outs 8 Frozen or intraoperative evaluations 8 Benign and/or high-risk lesions	
Plastic surgery	8 Reconstructive cases	
Imaging	8 Screening cases 8 Breast ultrasound 8 Diagnostic mammograms 8 Breast MRI	

Once the fellow has met minimum training requirements (Table 4.3), submits their minimum case operative logs into the database managed by ACGME, and completes a required Breast Fellows survey, they will be issued a Certificate of Completion granted by SSO. There is currently no separate board exam for breast surgical oncology at this time.

What to Look for in a Program

When deciding on a training program, consider a program that offers opportunity to experience benign as well as malignant breast disease. The majority of postgraduate fellows will likely be employed in a community-based hospital or medical center, with a smaller proportion at an academic institution. A study by Manahan et al. demonstrated that from a total of 843 members of ASBrS, 19.7% were in academic practice, vs. 80.2% who were either hospital employed, in a group practice, multi-specialty practice, or solo practice [1].

Breast conference is also a large component of your multidisciplinary training. As a requirement for the National Accreditation Program for Breast Centers (NAPBC), each breast center has to establish an interdisciplinary breast cancer conference on a regular basis. Expert surgeons, medical oncologists, radiation oncologists, pathologist, radiologists, geneticists, nurse practitioners, nurse navigators, physician assistants, research coordinators, and mental health professionals gather to discuss and develop a comprehensive plan for patient that is supported by evidence-based medicine and follow national guidelines.

Community Outreach

There are *tons* of community outreach opportunities during your fellowship year. Not only is it a fellowship requirement to engage in community outreach programs, it is to your benefit to become involved for several reasons. During our fellowship training, there were many open houses and forums for patients that were sponsored by various community outreach organizations, such as Susan G. Komen Foundation and Unite for Her. Some other support groups and outreach programs are The Amy Foundation, YSC Tour de Pink, Young Survival Coalition, Warriors in Pink, The Pink Fund, Lump to Laughter, I Will Survive, Inc., Avon Breast Health Outreach Program-Nueva Vida, Stupid Cancer (yes, this is an organization established in 2007 by young adults with cancer), and many more. It is crucial as a breast surgeon, not only to know how to perform the operations but to be aware of all aspects of breast cancer care, including what happens even after your patient is treated. Patients will expect you to be able to guide them not only medically and surgically but mentally, emotionally, physically, and sometimes even religiously. These community outreach programs provide an opportunity for that, as well as for you to familiarize yourself with lectures geared toward patients, families, and members of the medical community. This can also serve as a networking opportunity forming relationships that may lead to future referrals!

Lifestyle

As a breast surgeon, your schedule is more likely to be structured and manageable, compared to your general surgery colleagues and certainly from your residency days. There are, thankfully, few surgical emergencies related to breast care. The likelihood that you will need to worry about all those late night cases and early morning rounds will be slim. Even as a fellow, your schedule will be much more focused and structured. You will be able to tell your family members that you will be home for dinner and actually make it. You can tell your kids you will pick them up from school and not be lying! Lifestyle certainly should not be the *sole* reason you are pursuing breast surgery, but it is definitely a bonus.

As with all surgical specialties, the breast surgery world is a small one. Everyone knows someone who trained with someone, who now works with someone else. Work hard, be diligent, be passionate, be genuine, and be kind, to patients, colleagues, and your staff members. Everything else will follow. Good luck!!

References

1. Manahan E, et al. What is a breast surgeon worth? A salary survey of the American Society of Breast Surgeons. Ann Surg Oncol. 2015;22:3257–63.

Suggested Reading

Quinn McGlothin TD. Breast surgery as a specialized practice. Am J Surg. 2005;190(2):264–8.

Chapter 5
Burn Fellowship

Neha Amin

Application Process

A burn surgical fellowship is unique among the surgical fellowships. One is eligible to apply for a burn fellowship after completing at least 3 years of a general surgical residency. However, most programs do prefer postgraduate fellows. Applicants apply through individual programs as there is no unified match system. As of writing this chapter, there are currently 16 programs that have a burn surgery fellowship. Some programs have a built in critical care year along with the burn fellowship, but most will require you to apply for critical care separately if you would like an additional board certification.

Many programs can have internal candidates, and because of this, it can be difficult to know when to apply. There is no defined timeline for the burn fellowship application process. Some programs like you to apply during your fourth year, and some programs prefer your fifth year. It is personal preference to apply as early as possible or apply based on the timeline of your favorite programs. Keep in mind as there is no match system, the programs you apply to earlier will likely also have earlier deadlines for a response should they offer you a position. The easiest way to apply is to visit the website of each program that you are interested in. The website should have a contact email address who will be able to guide you through the application process.

Most programs are interested in past burn and critical care experience. Research experience, especially published, is a very strong addition to your CV. Make sure to attend and present, if possible, at national or regional burn conferences. The burn world is a small world, and it is very easy to meet and network at these conferences. Strong recommendation letters are very often brought up at interviews, and having this will definitely go a long way.

N. Amin, DO
Rowan University School of Osteopathic Medicine, Stratford, NJ, USA

© Springer International Publishing AG, part of Springer Nature 2018
K. Yoon-Flannery et al. (eds.), *A Surgeon's Path*,
https://doi.org/10.1007/978-3-319-78846-3_5

What to Look for in a Program

There is no unified organization that creates guidelines for the burn fellowship. The American Burn Association (ABA) certifies burn centers along with the American College of Surgeons with the ABA verification guidelines. However, they do not (currently) have any say in the development and education of the fellowship. Fellowships at ABA-verified centers are recommended as these centers must meet strict standards for organizational structure, personnel qualifications, facilities, and its resources and be up to date with treatments and goals.[1]

Another thing to consider is whether you would like an additional board certification along with your general surgery certification. A 1-year burn fellowship does not allow your eligibility to sit for anything further. Often, residents interested in burn fit into two categories—those also interested in pursuing critical care or those interested in pursuing plastic surgery fellowship. If you are considering critical care, it would be best to apply to a combined fellowship program or one that can help you in obtaining a critical care fellowship position for the following year. If you are interested in plastic surgery, look into a program that has a strong plastics team and presence in the burn unit. A good way to do this is to see whether the director of the burn unit is certified in one or the other.

It is also a good idea to consider the size of the burn unit, the level of the trauma center in the hospital, and the number of direct burn admissions per year. For a well-balanced education, you should seek a program that can firstly help you with your long-term interests and secondly a program that sees multiple different types of burn injuries. This should include thermal, chemical, electrical, friction, and radiation burns within the adult and pediatric populations. A good program will also have innovative ways to help treat large burns in the acute and chronic setting with reconstructive surgery, laser therapy, and specialized wound care.

Lifestyle

One of the best things about a burn fellowship is that it allows you to become specialized in many fields including wound care, critical care, and plastic surgery. You will often be able to tailor your life as you see fit with these multiple specializations. Burn fellows have gone on to either formally complete a plastic surgery fellowship, run burn units, be hospital surgicalists in a burn or acute care setting, continue locum tenens work in multiple critical care and burn hospitals, or even just focus on wound care in specialized wound care centers. You can be as busy as you want to be after this fellowship.

Applying for and participating in a burn fellowship are definitely a unique process. It can seem a bit daunting with no specific match system in the beginning.

[1] American Burn Association Verification [1].

However, having enthusiasm, a strong work ethic, and determination will get you far in this field.

References

1. American Burn Association Verification. Accessed from American Burn Association: http://ameriburn.org/quality-care/verification/. 2018, January.

Chapter 6
Colon and Rectal Surgery Fellowship

Mary T. O'Donnell and Nicole M. Saur

Introduction

Chances are you are surviving the rigors of a general surgery residency because you are one of the most talented, dedicated, and hardest working doctors in the hospital. Eighty percent of you will go on to do subspecialty training in a fellowship. Colon and rectal surgery (CRS) has become one of the most popular fellowships in recent years, filling 97–100% of nationwide spots for each of the last 5 years [1]. The number of CRS fellowships has increased from 36 in 2006 to 52 in 2016 to meet the demands of training the number of interested residents [1, 2]. Its popularity has led to a competitive application process, with an applicant per position available of 1.4:1 in 2016. A talent for using new surgical technology, an interest in diversity of disease processes and surgeries, and the ability to maintain work-life balance are some of the reasons doctors are drawn to CRS.

Variety Yet Expertise

The variety of disease processes in CRS is one of its main appeals. The colorectal (CR) surgeon must use his or her knowledge of disorders of the oncologic, dermatologic, and autoimmune nature on a daily basis. The CR surgeon must both be an expert proctologist and an oncologist, a balance between the sometimes light-hearted to the

M. T. O'Donnell, MD (✉)
Department of Colon and Rectal Surgery, Department of Surgery,
Ft. Belvoir Army Hospital, Arlington, VA, USA

Assistant Professor of Surgery, Uniformed Services University, Bethesda, MD, USA

N. M. Saur, MD
Division of Colon and Rectal Surgery, Department of Surgery, University of Pennsylvania,
Philadelphia, PA, USA

© Springer International Publishing AG, part of Springer Nature 2018   29
K. Yoon-Flannery et al. (eds.), *A Surgeon's Path*,
https://doi.org/10.1007/978-3-319-78846-3_6

most personal and serious aspects of life. As a cancer surgeon, the colorectal surgeon treats colon, rectal, and anal cancers to include adenocarcinoma, carcinoid tumors, GISTs, and melanoma in these areas. Colon cancer is the third most common cancer and second leading cause of cancer deaths in America. With nearly 140,000 new colon and rectal cancers estimated to be diagnosed in 2017, a malignancy cured exclusively with surgery requires an increasing number of specialists trained to do this [3]. Rectal cancer is treated in a multidisciplinary fashion and requires understanding of radiation and chemotherapy as adjuvant and neoadjuvant treatments. The increasing rates of rectal cancer among younger patients have led to interest in cancer genetics and the consideration for changes in screening tools [4]. Lastly, anal cancer is also treated with chemotherapy and radiation but requires the pattern recognition and physical exam skills of a colorectal surgeon to diagnose. The CR surgeon is truly an oncologic surgeon but, like many surgical oncologists, has specialized in a system of the body.

The CR surgeon must also be a keen dermatologist of the perianal area. The variety of dermatologic conditions affecting the anus requires experience with physical exam to differentiate precancerous lesions from benign conditions. The CR surgeon is often referred a patient with a concerning perianal finding or complaint regarding bowel movements, which must be parceled out to be concerning or benign. The diagnosis is often made on physical exam with a high index of suspicion based upon the history. Furthermore, surveillance after anal cancer treatment and in patients with anal dysplasia/HPV is a staple of the CR surgeon skill set in physical exam and diagnosis.

Inflammatory bowel disease (IBD) patients also compose much of the CR surgeon's practice. While Crohn's disease is mainly managed by gastroenterologists, when medications fail, the disease often becomes surgical. Often these patients are young and require multiple operations and an opportunity for longitudinal care. Ulcerative colitis is a disease that can be managed medically but ultimately is cured surgically.

Evolving Technology and Diversity of Skills

The constantly evolving field of colorectal surgery requires diversity in numerous skills including endoscopy and open, laparoscopic, and robotic surgery. The requirement of Fundamentals of Endoscopic Skills curriculum in general surgery residency highlights the importance of endoscopic skills in the surgeon's armamentarium. Surveillance of ileo-anal pouches and other surgical anastomoses by the surgeon maintains continuity of care. Large open cases are still common in CRS, while robotic surgery is taking hold in low pelvic surgery throughout the country. Anorectal cases are a mainstay of the CR surgeon's practice. Hemorrhoidectomy, anorectal fistula management, and fissure surgeries are usually short in duration but provide significant relief to patients.

Multidisciplinary Care

CR surgery practice builds relationships with different types of patients and multiple physician specialties within the hospital. Pilonidal disease can affect younger patients, while cancers can affect the elderly. Multidisciplinary care is achieved through coordination with urology (for stents or colovesicular fistulas), gynecology oncology (invasive rectal cancers or HPV-related perineal lesions), and plastic surgeons (flap creation within radiated fields).

Board Certification…In One Year!

The American Society of Colon and Rectal Surgeons (ASCRS) was founded in 1899, and the American Board of Colon and Rectal Surgery was founded in 1935. After fellowship, there is a written qualifying and oral certifying board examination, much like general surgery. The requirements to sit for the exam include performance of a specific number of anorectal, endoscopic, and large abdominal procedures – all of which are completed in a 1-year fellowship. The high-intensity training year is one of the shorter surgical fellowships in duration with the prestige of a board certification. Like the American College of Surgeons, ASCRS is very active nationally and can be a venue for those surgeons interested in changing policy.

Lifestyle

Most CR surgeons enjoy a better quality of life with work-life balance than other surgical subspecialties. The surgeon can be more or less busy depending on their stage of career, which can contribute to the longevity of a career as well. A number of CR surgeons practice well into their 70s, with an anorectal and endoscopic practice. The flexibility of the CR surgeon's practice allows for the ability to spend time on family life or academic pursuits of teaching or research. There are few true colon and rectal surgery emergencies as acute care surgery general surgeons often manage perforated diverticulitis and most small bowel obstructions. However, if you desire to have a practice of two full days of clinic and three full operating room days, you can achieve that as a CR surgeon. The number of people affected by cancer, IBD, and anorectal disorders is ample enough to support this schedule. Furthermore, if you desire to continue to practice general surgery, CRS is a specialty that can allow for that.

Broadened Practice

Depending on where you live in this country, CRS can be a niche or an addition skill. Less urban, rural areas of the United States are in need of general surgeons, and the CR surgeon who maintains board certification and still practices general surgery may be in high demand. Urban hospital systems tend to employ subspecialists, and the CR surgeon would likely practice exclusively CRS. The general surgery job market is interested in surgeons with colectomy experience, as this can make up a large part of a hospital's revenue. Fewer fellowships remain that require general surgery residency prior to application, and with the increasing desire for subspecialty training, there will be a shortage in general surgeons. The CR surgeon has the option to continue to practice general surgery and therefore may fill a future need for surgeons.

How to Get In!

Now that you have decided that colon and rectal surgery is the specialty for you, here are some tips to help you in the fellowship match.

Mentors

No matter the career you desire to pursue, mentorship is important to guiding, inspiring, and realizing that dream. Sound advice that we have received includes the need for more than one mentor. Specifically, you should try and have a senior and more junior mentor in a field of your interest. The senior mentor provides the long-term life example of where your career can be in 20 years from now, and his or her mentorship can help you make decisions now that can set you on a path toward your long-term goals. He/she is usually well-connected within ASCRS and can help you with opportunities to write book chapters, get involved in research projects, meet senior members of a potential practice to join, and understand what a career can achieve. A more junior mentor gives guidance and advice for the actions in the next 5 years that will allow you to manage the daily questions regarding a new surgery career. A junior mentor should be closer in age and training to you. He/she can help you choose a fellowship program, set up a practice, and even navigate early networking.

Early in training, it may be difficult to determine how to acquire a mentor. Sometimes it can be as easy as asking an attending, "can you mentor me?" What one has to understand is that the mentor-mentee relationship is actually symbiotic. Mentors are usually very interested in teaching and training but also rely on your burgeoning desire in the specialty to write/perform research or start projects that your mentor may have limited time to create. Usually, you have already developed a work relationship with an attending, and his/her career is, in some way, similar to the career you seek. Junior mentors can be more approachable due to their closeness in training and should be established early. Senior mentors can be sought through similar work relationships but also through junior mentors or other connections. Realize that the more senior a surgeon is, particularly in academic medicine, the busier he/she is, and approaching him/her with a mutual project may be a path toward mentorship.

While similar gender or background can be uniquely helpful in the selection of a mentor, it should not limit your choices. The unique challenges that you will face in your career can be understood and have been experienced in different ways by those surgeons that have trained before you. Therefore, it is to your advantage to continue to acquire mentors as your career progresses to suit its changing state.

Research

It is important to become involved in research in your desired specialty as it reflects an academic interest. General surgery residency has the benefit of allowing the resident to participate in projects of all subjects, and this demonstrates academic interest. Even if you do not desire a career in academic medicine, the involvement in research during training reflects highly on you in the eyes of fellowship programs. A clinical question related to CRS answered in a research project demonstrates an interest in the field and will provide a conversation piece in your fellowship interview.

Experience in the Field

Ensure you do a colorectal surgery rotation while in general surgery residency. It is important to know what the specialty entails on a day-to-day basis. These rotations will allow you to find mentors, imagine research projects, and determine if the specialty is for you. Enhanced recovery after surgery (ERAS) is an algorithm that gained popularity in the specialty of CRS and is an important change in the last few decades regarding postoperative care. Laparoscopy and open abdominal surgery are both integral to CRS, and interest in experience with both is necessary to train in the field.

Networking

Beyond your mentors, it is important to get to know other surgeons in the field, not only for fellowships but also for future job prospects. While the society has grown significantly, it is still a small enough community that many know each other.

Joining ASCRS will allow you to get notifications for the meeting, submit abstracts, and obtain information from the website. The meeting has resident-centered social events so that you can meet both peers interested in the specialty but also academic leaders in the field. Joining local and national surgical societies is to your advantage, especially if you trained at a smaller program. Join the American College of Surgeons, Society of Gastrointestinal and Endoscopic Surgeons (SAGES), and find out the local chapters of ASCRS or other specialty groups (Association of Women Surgeons, etc.). Connections you make at the meetings can lead to research opportunities, book chapter offerings, and fellowship interview opportunities!

Fellowship Application Timeline

The match for the CRS fellowships is through the National Resident Matching Program (NRMP), while the application process itself may be through the ERAS or the individual programs directly. The match usually opens mid-August, and the deadline for rank order list submission is usually in mid-October. The match result is usually released via email on November 1. More information on the application and timeline can be found at http://www.nrmp.org/fellowships/colon-and-rectal-surgery-match/.

In summary, colon and rectal surgery is a specialty with board certification, diversity of practice, and a manageable work-life balance. If you have an interest in the subject matter and surgeries involved in the CR surgeon's practice, it may be an interest to discuss with a surgeon mentor. Actively participate in your colorectal surgery rotation and, if desired, seek a CR surgeon mentor that can help guide you toward a career in colon and rectal surgery!

References

1. NRMP Match data @ http://www.nrmp.org/match-data/fellowship-match-data/
2. Birnbaum E. "Colorectal surgery" career development resource. Am J Surg. 2007;193:125–6.
3. American Cancer Society Key Statistics @ https://www.cancer.org/cancer/colon-rectal-cancer/about/key-statistics.html and https://cancerstatisticscenter.cancer.org/#/
4. Siegel RL, Fedewa SA, Anderson WF, Miller KD, Ma J, Rosenberg PS, Jemal A. Colorectal cancer incidence patterns in the United States, 1974-2013. J Natl Cancer Inst. 2017;109(8). https://doi.org/10.1093/jnci/djw322.

Chapter 7
Complex General Surgical Oncology Fellowship

Shanel B. Bhagwandin and Devin C. Flaherty

Introduction

Surgical oncology is a challenging surgical subspecialty, and general surgery trainees can only truly appreciate the professional demands required of a surgical oncologist through ongoing exposure and postgraduate fellowship training. A surgical oncologist is a highly specialized surgeon who is not only trained in the complex surgical management of malignancies but is also an integral member of a patient's multidisciplinary treatment team that serves to manage and optimize the delivery of cancer care. Recognizing that cancer knows no bounds and new advances in the field of oncology are continually being applied, a surgical oncologist must efficiently address all aspects of a patient's oncologic treatment in order to provide a personalized treatment plan. During general surgery training, mentorship from surgical oncologists allows residents to recognize the rewards and challenges this specialty provides. What truly differentiates complex general surgical oncology from other surgical specialties is the training in oncologic operations fellows receive, as well as collaborative multidisciplinary treatment planning in a complex patient population.

S. B. Bhagwandin, DO, MPH (✉)
Division of Surgical Oncology, Department of Surgery, The Icahn School of Medicine at Mount Sinai, New York, NY, USA

Surgical Oncology and Hepatopancreatobiliary Surgery, Jupiter Medical Center/Jupiter Medical Specialists, Jupiter, FL, USA
e-mail: Shanel.bhagwandin@mountsinai.org

D. C. Flaherty, DO, PhD, FACOS
Valley Health Surgical Oncology, Winchester, VA, USA

© Springer International Publishing AG, part of Springer Nature 2018
K. Yoon-Flannery et al. (eds.), *A Surgeon's Path*,
https://doi.org/10.1007/978-3-319-78846-3_7

The Path to Fellowship

A resident's awareness of surgical oncology typically begins in the operating room through observation and participation in complex oncology cases. One can't help but acknowledge the advanced surgical skills a surgical oncologist must possess to successfully operate in a surgical field marred by the invasive nature of cancer. Further interest may be spurred on the wards, as a surgical oncologist must have a clinical acumen beyond what may be perceived as the "scope" of their specialty. Should a trainee have the privilege of participating in a surgical oncologist's clinic, they will quickly recognize the increased time spent with patients and their families as they grapple with a diagnosis, their mortality, and potentially extensive surgical procedures. As with any surgical specialty, the procedures a surgical oncologist performs can be rife with complications. Unique to surgical oncology, these complications may delay further oncologic therapy or have lasting effects on a patient's quality of life. It is important that a cancer patient is fully educated on the course of their care. Finally, multidisciplinary conferences such as tumor boards expose trainees to a very important role surgical oncologists fulfill—being part of a multidisciplinary treatment team. Residents interested in surgical oncology often look forward to attending these conferences in order to observe and sometimes be part of the interaction between specialists such as medical oncologists, radiation oncologists, gastroenterologists, pathologist, radiologist, palliative care practitioners, nurses, social workers, and of course, surgical oncologists. This collaborative approach to cancer care resounds in those interested in surgical oncology, and it is through an opportunity to discuss recommended treatment regiments that trainees bound for a career in surgical oncology realize that a comprehensive approach to their patient's cancer care is what they seek.

Should a resident decide to pursue a career in surgical oncology, it is important to nurture the relationships developed with training surgical oncologists. These surgeons can act as mentors and can greatly assist a resident with preparations for fellowship application. Many mentors may advise taking time off from general surgery training to pursue basic science or clinical research projects that will help make a candidate's application more well-rounded. Most surgical oncology fellowship applicants have an established foundation in research, affording them research presentations at regional and/or national meetings and publication of their research in scientific journals. Having a passion for research is important for applicants as the surgeon-scientist embraces the true essence of surgical oncology, that being technical excellence in the operating room and continued advancement in field of cancer. Keeping this in mind, there is no one formula for success, and many applicants successfully match into a surgical oncology fellowship having participated only in research conducted during their 5 years of general surgery training. Many general surgery programs offer concurrent degrees in other healthcare specialties such as Master of Public Health (MPH), which is also favorably looked upon by application committees.

Fellowship Application

Surgical oncology as a fellowship has undergone a major transformation over the last 5 years. Fellows in complex general surgical oncology fellowships now have the opportunity to be board certified, as the Accreditation Council for Graduate Medical Education (ACGME) now accredits a multitude training programs throughout the United States. Graduates from the graduating fellow class of 2014 were the first fellows eligible to sit for the complex general surgical oncology boards, and board certification is not being extended retroactively to any previous trainees in surgical oncology. Previously, surgical oncology was a nonaccredited fellowship sponsored by the Society of Surgical Oncology (SSO). The number of applicants to complex general surgical oncology fellowship programs has been steadily increasing, and greater than 50% of applicants typically do not match. Receiving an interview by a fellowship program is significant and generally required in order to attain a fellowship position. Interviews are fairly benign as training programs seek mainly to get to know the applicant that is well supported by their accomplishments and letters of recommendation.

Competitive applicants applying to a large number of fellowships may be offered an interview at 10–15 programs. Some programs may interview anywhere from 8 candidates for one fellowship position, while others may interview between 30 and 40 candidates over two separate dates for a variety of positions. After the interview, interested programs may reach out to an applicant to clarify the applicants' career goals and interests and to answer any final questions.

The interview trail offers a unique setting that allows applicants to forge lasting relationships with each other as most applicants are traveling to the same cities for the same interviews. After the match and matriculation into fellowship, the Society of Surgical Oncology Annual Cancer Symposium is often a site for informal interview class reunions. As applicants learn more and more about their colleagues on the interview trail, they will appreciate the similarities and differences in each other's applications. These interactions may help an applicant identify what a specific program is looking for in a fellowship candidate and ultimately assist an applicant determine their rank list.

Fellowship

Congratulations! You matched and are officially a complex general surgical oncology fellow. While each fellowship program varies with regard to autonomy, case volume, and quality of life, there are a few basic tenets that a fellow should adhere to in order to make their fellowship a success. Most fellowship programs will have an apprenticeship model where a fellow will spend a set amount of time with either one or a group of surgical oncologists in a disease-specific area. Alternatively, some programs will utilize a single service that covers the breadth of complex general surgical oncology. A fellow's rotation through each surgical oncology service will afford training in the management of various malignancies, operations, as well as the accompanying perioperative management. While rotating on different services, a fellow should take note of the variety of clinical approaches to surgical planning, operative techniques, and overall cancer care. A fellow should appreciate that their fellowship is likely at a high-volume cancer center that affords many resources for cancer care, and this experience is likely not representative of the way most cancer care is delivered throughout the country.

Fellow case volume, case complexity, and autonomy in the operating room will increase as a fellow progresses through fellowship. The surgical oncologists a fellow operates under will not only train the fellow in the oncological principles underlying surgical resections but will also teach safe surgical techniques. Also critical to the training of a surgical oncologist is a constant focus on preoperative decision-making and multidisciplinary management of each patient before and after surgery. Multidisciplinary conferences are an integral component of a fellow's training as the fellow will have the responsibilities of presenting cases and proposing management strategies that adhere to supporting literature and known standards of care. Multidisciplinary care is at the foundation of all surgical oncology trainings, and understanding how to make collaborative decisions will advance a fellow's training and serve their patients well.

As a fellow matures during fellowship, he or she must continually challenge himself or herself to learn as much as possible during their short training. A trainee finally finds himself or herself in a position where one can focus on specific areas of interest, and continued reading and case preparation are essential. Several months of fellowship will be spent on nonsurgical rotations such as medical oncology, radiation oncology, pathology, genetics, etc. These rotations offer an opportunity to gain multidisciplinary knowledge. Further, these rotations often afford a fellow more time for research activities ensuring one is able to stay ahead of national and regional meeting deadlines. Some fellows will choose to spend time in the lab, and balancing that with clinical responsibilities may be difficult. There are programs that offer an optional third year of training in order to complete a more advance research project.

Job Search

As a fellow begins their second year of fellowship, interests in an area of surgical oncology should be established as well as the desired practice environment (i.e., academic versus community/private practice). These interests should be discussed regularly with the Fellowship Program Director and other mentors, as they will be a graduate's biggest advocates when applying for a position. The application process for a surgical oncology position is typically initiated in the fall/winter of a fellow's second year. Resources for complex general surgical oncology jobs include society websites, community job-search forums, and word of mouth. Open junior faculty positions at an academic institution may be discovered through conversations at annual meetings or by inquiry on an applicant's behalf by a mentor.

As previously mentioned, there is variation in surgical oncology training. A fellow's first job will likely continue to provide on-the-job training as they navigate the complex waters of surgical oncology attendingship. For example, a graduate may require advanced laparoscopic or endoscopic skills that were not nurtured in fellowship necessitating continued medical education courses and mentorship from other surgical oncologists. Further, treatment approaches toward certain malignancies and the scope of practice of certain subspecialties may vary depending on the area of the country one is practicing. It is important to recognize these potential opportunities or obstacles when interviewing for a first job.

Board Certification

The American Board of Surgery certifies complex general surgical oncology candidates completing a 2-year or 3-year ACGME-accredited complex general surgical oncology fellowship after passing both a written and an oral exam. Fellows must be certified by the American Board of Surgery in general surgery prior to sitting for their complex general surgical oncology boards. The written examination is typically completed in the fall following graduation from fellowship. The oral examination is offered once a year (typically in January or February) in a variety of cities across the United States. Examination pass rates are easily referenced online. Currently, there are ongoing efforts by the Surgical Council on Resident Education (SCORE) to create a complex general surgical oncology board preparation curriculum.

Conclusions

Complex general surgical oncology fellowship is a unique and challenging post-residency surgical training curriculum. To find success, one requires strong mentorship and a zest for both surgery and research. With board certification now offered, it is expected that complex general surgical oncology fellowship positions will continue to be competitively pursued.

Suggested Reading

Berman RS, Weigel RJ. Training and certification of the surgical oncologist. Chin Clin Oncol. 2014;3:45.
Tyler DS, Michelassi F. Finish line or beginning? Welcome the new board-certified surgical oncologists. Ann Surg Oncol. 2016;23:1403–8.
Wyld L, Audisio RA, Poston GJ. The evolution of cancer surgery and future perspectives. Nat Rev Clin Oncol. 2015;12:115–24.

Chapter 8
Vascular Surgery Fellowship

Holly Graves

Overview

Vascular surgery encompasses a broad range of pathologies as well as operative and endovascular procedures. Vascular surgery practices range from large academic tertiary care centers to private practices with office-based procedures, wound care, and dialysis access management. The field is constantly evolving as new technologies and devices are introduced. Vascular surgery offers the opportunity to treat a variety of patients, ranging from the pediatric population to extremely sick patients with multiple comorbidities. Patients with vascular conditions are often followed for long periods of time which can be a satisfying form of patient care. Surgeons choose vascular surgery for many reasons, and most are ultimately very satisfied with their career.

Application Process

There are three ways to pursue vascular training: the newly formed integrated vascular surgery track (0 + 5), the traditional vascular fellowship track (5 + 2), and the Early Specialization Program (ESP) track (4 + 2), which allows the chief year to be used as the first year of vascular surgery training. This is available only in programs with ESP accreditation and is still consisted of 2 years of dedicated vascular training. This chapter will focus on the *traditional vascular fellowship track (5 + 2)*. This pathway requires completion of 5 years of general surgery training and allows for board certification in general surgery and vascular surgery. Requirements for general surgery board certification are program dependent; however, most vascular

H. Graves, MD
Jefferson Health New Jersey, Voorhees, NJ, USA
e-mail: h.graves@kennedyhealth.org

© Springer International Publishing AG, part of Springer Nature 2018
K. Yoon-Flannery et al. (eds.), *A Surgeon's Path*,
https://doi.org/10.1007/978-3-319-78846-3_8

surgery fellowships recommend general surgery board certification. The timing of fellowship has recently changed in that fellowship begins in the August of the year that general surgery residency is completed. The general surgery written boards are now offered in the July of that same graduating year.

Residents typically apply for the vascular surgery fellowship in February of their fourth clinical year of general surgery training. The traditional application process is through the Electronic Residency Application Service (ERAS). The vascular surgery match is announced that following May. The number of vascular surgery fellowship positions offered varies from year to year depending on which programs decide to participate in the match and how many candidates they are accepting. Candidates may apply to as many or as few programs as they choose, and this number strongly varies. The application process can become expensive as the application fee itself as well as the interview accommodations are covered by the fellowship candidate.

Considerations

When applying to a fellowship, one needs to consider both the quality of training and quality of life. Not all programs are intense as others, and programs range from more of a community-based practice to a large tertiary care facility. The focus of one program may be "bread and butter" vascular procedures, whereas another program may be focused on aortic interventions. Though it is important to choose a program based off of one's interest, it is important to be broadly trained. Also, if one does train at a smaller community hospital, it is not impossible to find a career opportunity at a large academic institution and vice versa.

There are many questions to consider when applying and interviewing at various programs. It is important to ask about the volume and type of procedures being performed by the fellows. It is just as crucial to know the strengths and weaknesses of each program in terms of the number of procedures being done. Inquire about the amount of open versus endovascular procedures, especially regarding aortic work, as open abdominal aortic aneurysm repairs are being done less frequently with the new endovascular technologies. Also, inquire about the breakdown of endovascular procedures, specifically what procedures and how many of the procedures are being done by interventional cardiology and radiology. Make sure the program has some trauma exposure. When touring the facilities, get an idea of what is available to the fellows, for example, are most endovascular procedures being done with a c-arm or is there a hybrid room? Also try to get an idea of how much the fellow is participating in the case and if the graduating fellows feel competent to perform procedures on their own as an attending. Lastly make sure the program offers ample office hour exposure as this is a large part of a vascular surgery practice as an attending.

Apart from the vascular training itself, one must consider quality of life. When talking with fellows, ask them to describe a typical day in terms of how many hours they work and what the typical call schedule includes – especially nighttime emergencies. Are there junior residents and/or mid-level providers on the service to help with patient care, and most importantly, are the fellows happy overall? It is also important to get an idea of the living situation for the fellows, such as the safety of the hospital and cost of living. Some programs cover multiple hospitals; therefore, a car may be required. It is important to consider all of these facts as a period of 2 years is a long time to be miserable.

Vascular Lab

Vascular laboratory interpreting skills are a crucial part of vascular training. Depending of the type of practice one chooses, reading vascular lab studies can be a substantial part of one's practice. Vascular board certification now requires passing the Physicians' Vascular Interpretation (PVI) exam and Registered Physician in Vascular Interpretation (RPVI) certification before being able to sit for the vascular boards. Eligibility for the PVI exam requires documentation of reviewing 500 vascular lab studies broken down into various categories, such as aortic, peripheral arterial, carotid, venous, and so forth. The PVI exam is offered twice a year, usually in September to October (register June to August) and March to April (register December to March). Most fellows opt to take the exam their second year of fellowship.

Research

The amount of time allotted for vascular research is program dependent. Research is usually more heavily emphasized in academic programs, though this is not always the case. A research background is not necessarily required to apply to vascular fellowship, though it is looked upon highly, even if the research was not necessarily vascular-based. Most fellowships offer opportunities to attend and present at various conferences, both locally and nationally. Funding and time allotted for such opportunities are program dependent and should be something you consider asking during your interviews.

Boards

The Vascular Surgery Qualifying Exam is now offered in September. If one passes the qualifying exam, one is invited to sit for the Vascular Surgery Certifying Exam that following May. Both exams are offered once yearly. Once the qualifying exam is passed, the candidate has three opportunities to pass the oral boards before remedial action is taken.

Getting a Job

Most fellows begin applying for jobs at the beginning of their second year of fellow-ship. Job opportunities can be found on various vascular society websites and meet-ings, local healthcare job fairs and recruiters, as well as by word of mouth. There is a wide range of vascular surgery attending salaries depending on location and type of practice one chooses.

Resources

American Board of Surgery. http://www.absurgery.org
American Registry for Diagnostic Medical Sonography. http://www.ARDMS.org
Electronic Residency Application Service. http://www.AAMC.org/services/ERAS
Society for Vascular Surgery. http://www.vascular.org

Chapter 9
Minimally Invasive Surgery Fellowship

Roshin Thomas and Stefanie Haynes

Application Process

The minimally invasive surgery (MIS) fellowship is a 1-year fellowship. It is open to anyone who is board eligible/certified in general surgery. Some exceptions may be possible; however they are determined by the fellowship program director. Applicants apply through the Fellowship Council, which offers programs that are focused in minimally invasive surgery, hepatobiliary, bariatric surgery, and advanced endoscopy. Applicants may choose whether they want to apply to programs focused on a certain specialty or programs that offer all of these options. It is important to note that the Fellowship Council also offers information and applications to those applying for non-ACGME thoracic and colorectal fellowships.

The Fellowship Council has a very comprehensive website detailing all the pre-requisites necessary for the application process. Candidates can apply at any point after the completion of their PGY 3 or follow a more traditional timeline and apply during the PGY 4. The application process for this current year opens on December 4, 2018, and closes on February 13, 2019. After this date, no further applications will be accepted. Interviews are offered in a rolling basis. Of course, the earlier one applies, the more potential interviews one may achieve. The programs will continue to grant interviews to applicants until March 16, 2019, and the interview season typically lasts through the month of May. Most programs will offer two or three interview dates for which you can decide which date works best for your schedule. For the majority of participating programs, the applicants will compete for one fellow position; however some programs offer 2–3 positions.

R. Thomas, DO (✉)
Rowan University School of Osteopathic Medicine, Stratford, NJ, USA

S. Haynes, DO
Philadelphia College of Osteopathic Medicine, Philadelphia, PA, USA

© Springer International Publishing AG, part of Springer Nature 2018
K. Yoon-Flannery et al. (eds.), *A Surgeon's Path*,
https://doi.org/10.1007/978-3-319-78846-3_9

After all of the traveling and shaking hands, the rank list is finally due on May 24, 2019. The results of the match are posted on two separate days. On June 12 at 12:00 pm noon, the applicant will learn whether they have matched into a program. If the answer is yes, the applicant will wait for 24 h until June 13 with the destination of match is announced. If the answer is no, the applicant will need to enter the scramble process. Applicants can then go onto the Fellowship Council website and look for the programs that have available spots. At this time the applicant will call the available programs, complete phone interviews, and possibly match into a program.

As with medical school and residency, to ensure a stress-free match process, one must start gathering material for the application process as soon as possible. The requirements that often take a long time are logging cases and requesting letters of recommendation. You will need a minimum of three (maximum of five) letters. This is the rate – limiting step of the process as you may assume that your attending surgeons are busy. As soon as one decides to apply to MIS fellowship, start requesting and collecting all of your letters of recommendation.

How can one be a strong candidate, you ask? As with previous applications, board and in-service exams weigh heavily on the examiners. However, this is not the only thing that is taken into account. Strong letters of recommendations or a phone call from a reputable surgeon can go a long way, so do not be afraid to ask for help. Just remember, if you are thinking of doing it, there is someone out there who has already done it. To strengthen your application, it also helps to be part of the American College of Surgeons (ACS), Society of American Gastrointestinal and Endoscopic Surgeons (SAGES), and/or the American Society of Bariatric and Metabolic Surgeons (ASMBS). Acceptance into these societies requires further letters of recommendation from your program director and an active member of this society. SAGES offers a resident membership which does not require an application fee. It also is helpful to attend one of these annual clinical assembly conferences if able. This is a great opportunity to meet program directors from various programs, not to mention gives you a topic to talk about during your interview. Lastly, research is another strong component to add to your application. Focus on ways to separate yourself from the hundreds of other applicants.

Applicants can contact the Fellowship Council office with any questions at 310-437-0555 or email info@fellowshipcouncil.org.

Fees

Applications fees are as follows:

$200 for the first 20 fellowship programs
$100 per each additional 10 fellowship programs thereafter

Components of Training

Fellows are trained to become competent in six major areas during their fellowship year:

(a) Promoting health care that is patient centered, reflecting compassion and effective toward the treatment of their problems.
(b) Demonstrate excellent dexterity and show that they are capable of developing and executing plans for patient care
(c) Develop their knowledge about established and evolving issues in biomedical and clinical sciences.
(d) Develop interpersonal and communication skills among patients, patient family members as well as other health professionals.
(e) Professionalism, commitment toward patient care, and maintaining and holing oneself to high ethical standards.
(f) Systems-based practice such as learning to be cost-effective, learning risk-benefit analysis, and understanding the importance of other specialists in patient care.

What to Look for in a Program

As mentioned previously, the Fellowship Council showcases a variety of programs with specific areas of focus. The applicant must decide whether they want a program that is more geared toward bariatric surgery versus hepato-pancreaticobiliary or endoscopy. With bariatric-focused fellowships, it is important to note whether these programs are able to obtain at least the minimum number of cases that the ASMBS has deemed as the number to be certified. There are programs in which the fellow will function as junior attending surgeons during their year in fellowship. This means that the applicant is able to practice as an independent general surgeon and take general surgery call individually. If you want more endoscopy experience, there are also programs that focus on this as well. Each program has a detailed case log of prior fellows completed operations, which the applicant can refer to before deciding if they would like to train there or not.

What Can You Do with this Fellowship?

After completion of a minimally invasive fellowship, you will have the option of practicing as a general surgeon, bariatric surgeon, or endoscopic specialized surgeon. This means that you can move toward a more elective practice, if that is your goal. However, if you would like to continue practicing general surgery, this fellowship is an advanced extension of the newest technology in general surgery. This is maybe an ideal fellowship for someone who loves general surgery but also would like to perfect their laparoscopic skills and ultimately benefit your patients in the end!

As with everything in life, it is all about how much you are willing to put into the application process. A great work ethic and a solid personality can take you a long way. A well-rounded applicant with a strong handshake is your key to success! Good luck and Godspeed!

Resources

Fellowship Programs. (2018). https://fellowshipcouncil.org/fellowship-programs/

Chapter 10
Plastic Surgery Fellowship

Sarah N. Bishop and Nakul Rao

Introduction

There are two main pathways to obtain training in plastic surgery: the integrated and the independent model. The integrated model is a residency and matches mainly fourth year medical students. The independent model is the traditional model and has two options. The first option consists of the completion of 3 years of clinical general surgery training followed by 3 years of plastic surgery training. This option is only feasible if the general surgery training and plastic surgery training are completed at the same institution. The second option can be utilized by those who have completed formal training and are board eligible/board certified in either general surgery, otolaryngology, neurosurgery, orthopedic surgery, urology, or oral and maxillofacial surgery. Most residents applying are PGY4 general surgery residents matching for fellowships to begin at the completion of their chief/PGY5. However, residents from other training pathways are generally viewed favorably and have a different skill set to offer and sell. The second option is the most common pathway and what we will focus on mainly in this chapter.

S. N. Bishop, MD (✉)
Division of Plastic and Reconstructive Surgery, Mayo Clinic, Rochester, MN, USA
e-mail: Bishop.sarah1@mayo.edu

N. Rao, MD
Department of Surgery, Drexel University College of Medicine, Philadelphia, PA, USA

© Springer International Publishing AG, part of Springer Nature 2018
K. Yoon-Flannery et al. (eds.), *A Surgeon's Path*,
https://doi.org/10.1007/978-3-319-78846-3_10

Application Process

The matching process for residents matching into a plastic surgery fellowship is performed through the San Francisco Match (SF Match). This is a matching service that matches several different residencies and fellowships. All of the basic information on matching into a plastics fellowship is available at http://sfmatch.org/. On the home page, you can select "Specialties," and then under Residencies, select "Plastics." Although technically this will be a fellowship, many consider plastics to be considered more like residency training as the scope of the material is so different from general surgery. When deciding to go into a plastics fellowship, one must be prepared to "be an intern again." Unlike other fellowships off of general surgery, such as minimally invasive surgery (MIS) or trauma, where residents have had extensive training, plastic surgery truly is a new skill set with completely new information. Thus, the terms residents/fellows or residency/fellowships will often be used interchangeably at certain programs.

To have a complete application for the SF Match, several things need to be accomplished via the Central Application Service (CAS). This is a basic online application completed through the SF Match. After completing the online application, you will need to upload the following items to have a complete application:

(a) Medical school transcripts
(b) USMLE scores or ECFMG (if international graduate)
(c) Photograph
(d) Three letters of reference
(e) Photocopy of American Board of Plastic Surgery Resident Registration and Evaluation of Training Form Confirmation Letter
(f) Physician Information Profile requested from Federation Credentials Verification Service (FCVS) available at http://www.fsmb.org

At least one of the recommendation letters should be from a plastic surgeon, preferably the Chair of Plastic Surgery at your current program. You should waive your right to see their letters. You will also be required to detail every rotation, including research, and vacation time for all years of your training on your application. You will also need to submit the rotations you will be taking in your final year of training which you have not completed yet. If you do not know what your schedule will be, use a current chief's schedule.

This application process can take several months to complete. You should anticipate 6 months to complete the entire process. You will also be given the option of where to send your Physician Information Profile on your application. You should select that your profile be sent directly to the SF Match. You can also select that the profile be sent to yourself. However, sending the profile to SF Match will expedite SF Match ultimately receiving your profile.

The rate-limiting step in completing a timely application is the evaluation of training letter and a completed FCVS. Ideally these should be started in the spring prior to submitting your completed application in the fall. For example, start FCVS and training letter in spring 2017; submit completed application through the SF Match in fall 2017, interviews in winter/spring 2018, and with a Match Day in May 2018 for the training to begin in July 2019.

A timeline is given within the SF Match website which sites November as a "deadline" for application. However, programs will look at applications at different times. The safest is to have the application completed by the end of September or early October.

Interviews

You will be notified of an interview by either email or through messages from the SF Match. If you have given more than one email through the SF Match, then you should check all of your email accounts for interview offers. Have alerts on your phone for email updates as interview offers will usually have 1–4 possible dates, which are first come first serve. Call and schedule your interview immediately to secure your preferred date. You can call programs ahead of time to find out when they are interviewing so that you keep those dates open for programs that you are really interested in.

Remember that you will meet lifelong friends on the interview trail. Although you are in competition with each other, this should not preclude you from being cordial and from developing lasting friendships.

The key is to know your application thoroughly and to be yourself. Those involved in plastic surgery are often creative and artistic. If you have a special talent, make it known on your application but be prepared to discuss or even demonstrate. Do not lie to impress. Rarely interviewers may ask you to draw something or sculpt something to demonstrate your ability to think three-dimensionally. Having an artistic ability is by no means a prerequisite but can help for the programs that may be interested.

Expense

The interviewing process can be extremely expensive and time consuming, but there are ways to maximize your budget and time. Use your frequent flyer miles. If you stick to one airline as much as possible, you can often get free upgrades and priority check in. Take the initial time to do a pre-TSA check in, which involves an online application and a fingerprinting appointment. After this process is complete, you will be able to go through security expeditiously. You can use a phone app to reserve rental cars. Renting a car is usually cheaper than a taxi or other car services, and phone apps tend to offer better deals than online. You should also try to travel with carry-on luggage only. This is much cheaper and faster and avoids the disaster of the airline losing your luggage and you not having a suit to wear to your interview.

During our interview process, one of our colleagues had unfortunately gotten his luggage lost during his flight. He had no way to obtain a suit for the interview, which was due to start at 6 am. He ended up going to the interview with various borrowed pieces from his fellow interviewees! Don't let this happen to you.

The fellowship programs will often give you a recommendation for a hotel to stay with a discount. Make sure to use hotel rewards if applicable. Book as soon as you have confirmed your interview date.

Match

You will submit your rank list 1 week before you obtain your results through the SF Match. Refer to the SF Match for the exact dates of your year. On your Match Day, you will log in to the SF Match and your account to obtain your results.

If you have matched, congratulations! If unfortunately you do not match, there will be vacancies listed for those programs with open spots. Be aggressive when trying to secure a position if you did not match.

Fellowship

You will begin fellowship the following year after your match. Try as much as possible to prepare during your chief year. The more prepared you are, the less daunting it will be starting an entirely different field. You do not need to exhaustively prepare, but if you are able to read through Grabb and Smiths and/or Janis' *Essentials of Plastic Surgery*, this will help greatly. There is nothing more terrifying than covering your first busy hand/face/plastics call when you are ill prepared.

Many struggle with beginning a new specialty and having to start over. It is very difficult to go from being a chief resident to now becoming an intern again. This is a difficult transition for everyone but it will ultimately pass if you stick with it.

Programs will either be entirely made of fellows of a combination of integrated and independent residents. Both offer pros/cons. For those independent-only programs, when you start you will truly be the intern. However, everyone will be similarly trained to you, and you will be on an equal playing field. For those in the integrated/independent programs, you will be starting out as a PGY6; however, some programs will essentially consider you to be a PGY4 (the equivalent year for an integrated resident). You will not truly be considered an intern, but you will be compared to integrated residents who have spent 3 more years in plastic surgery training than you have. It can be quite difficult to realize that on day 1 of your training, you are far behind in your plastic surgery knowledge than a PGY2 or even PGY1. However, in general your overall technical skills and clinical acumen will make up for this. Work hard to improve your plastic surgery knowledge so that you can catch up and hopefully surpass!

Research

Research is an important aspect of obtaining a plastics fellowship. Realize that residents applying for integrated residencies have often spent years in research in order to be competitive enough to apply for a plastics residency straight out of medical school. Independent residents are not generally expected to have the same amount of research. However, for elite positions research is key, and ultimately independents will be competing with integrated residents for subspecialty fellowships where research can be a deciding factor.

Subspecialty Fellowships

After plastics fellowship you can go onto practice or obtain further subspecializations, mostly through matching services. Subspecialties include microsurgery, craniofacial, hand, aesthetics, and head and neck fellowships.

Resources

American Council of Academic Plastic Surgeons (ACAPS). http://www.acaplastic-surgeons.org
Federation Credentials Verification Service. http://www.fsmb.org
Plastic Surgery Information Service. http://plasticsurgery.org
PRS Match. https://sites.google.com/site/prsmatch/
San Francisco Match. https://sfmatch.org
The American Board of Plastic Surgery. https://abplasticsurgery.org

Chapter 11
Transplant Fellowship

David P. St. Michel

Introduction

After years of study, hard work, and missing time with loved ones, you have decided to continue this path and pursue a fellowship in transplant surgery. You have chosen a challenging and time-consuming career that allows you to provide care to some of the sickest patients you could ever encounter. You will have incredibly difficult experiences with patients you are unable to help but be rewarded with the amazing sense of accomplishment when your patients are able to return to living full and meaningful lives.

The purpose of this chapter is to provide a base of information about the application process, share some of my experiences as a resident who recently participated in the match, and hopefully alleviate some of the stress that comes along with entering this field. Transplant surgery is a relatively young, evolving specialty comprised of a small committed group of surgeons, medical specialists, and other professionals. Many residents may not have had extensive experience in the field, often consisting of a few rotations, and frequently may not have had a close mentor available to help guide them through the process. My hope is that these few pages can help you on the path to entering this specialty.

D. P. St. Michel, DO, MPH
Division of Transplant Surgery, University of Maryland School of Medicine,
Baltimore, MD, USA
e-mail: David.stmichel@nv.touro.edu

© Springer International Publishing AG, part of Springer Nature 2018
K. Yoon-Flannery et al. (eds.), *A Surgeon's Path*,
https://doi.org/10.1007/978-3-319-78846-3_11

Application

Transplant fellowships are accredited by the American Society of Transplant Surgeons (ASTS). The website should be a starting point for your applications process. On it you will find a timeline of events for the match, which typically opens in March and has a rank list close date at the end of May. Match day is in June of your fourth year. The match is orchestrated through the National Resident Matching Program (NRMP) system used for the residency match, but all programs have their own requirements and applications that must be completed as well. Interviews will be between January and April of your PGY-4. I would recommend having your applications completed in early December.

As you did for residency applications, start compiling your transcripts and putting together your CV. While having transplant-dedicated research is desirable, you can demonstrate that you will be productive during your fellowship by presenting and publishing work in any surgical field. Having several projects on your CV will strengthen your application, so start finishing those case reports and studies that have stalled as early as possible.

Most programs require three letters of recommendation—one from your Residency Program Director and two from other attendings, though this can vary. Ask for these months in advance. Most attendings are very busy - don't hesitate to remind them of upcoming due dates. Letters from transplant surgeons are not required. A solid recommendation from a bariatric surgeon you have worked extensively with may be more meaningful than a form letter from a transplant surgeon with whom you scrubbed three cases. If you have the opportunity to work with a transplant surgeon, make the most of it. Volunteer to do the midnight donor operations, assist with backbench preparation of the organs in cases that you aren't covering, and know the pre- and post-transplant patients inside and out. Transplant centers have listing meetings frequently and generally residents are welcome to attend. Again, transplant surgery is a small community and the attendings you are interviewing with may well know the surgeon who is writing you a letter of recommendation.

Personal statements are always difficult to write. They should be brief (1 page) and express why you desire this career and why you will excel. A trusted and critical person should review this and offer suggestions. The message of my statement remained the same, but after several versions, the final product was far superior because of this helpful, and sometimes painful, feedback.

The ASTS website provides a list of all accredited programs, what certifications they offer and contact information. Use this as a starting point for determining where you would like to apply. For the 2016 match, there were 58 programs, but each program may offer certification in different procedures. Transplant fellowships are 2 years in length, and for accreditation a program must perform a minimum number of transplantations yearly for the following organs: 60 for kidney, 50 for liver, 20 for pancreas, and 10 for intestinal transplantation. The ASTS also accredits programs for hepatobiliary (HB) and hepato-pancreatico-biliary (HPB) training, with a case volume of 50 cases (subdivided by procedure) required yearly. For a fellow to receive a certificate in these procedures, they must be the principal operator for 40 renal transplants, 45 hepatic transplants, 15 pancreas transplants, 10 intestinal transplants, 35 HB cases, and 50 HPB cases (American Society of Transplant Surgeons http://www.asts.org).

Programs may be accredited in one, two, or more of these surgeries. Most transplant centers offer training in all of these (except intestine) and you will likely get exposure to liver transplants even at programs that are not accredited to offer that certification. You can even perform these transplants if granted privileges as an attending at your institution without the certificate. Not obtaining a certificate may, however, preclude you from holding certain leadership positions (i.e., Program Director) in the future. Once you have decided in which organs you would like to be certified, two useful sources are the Organ Procurement and Transplantation Network (OPTN) and the Scientific Registry of Transplant Recipients (SRTR). Both websites provide detailed information about the transplants performed at individual institutions. OPTN provides yearly volume data on each center and the types of transplants performed, while the SRTR provides 18-month detailed reports on volume, institutional outcomes compared to expected outcomes, waitlist information, and other data. OPTN data is generally close to real time, whereas SRTR is updated with each new report. Familiarize yourself with both of these sites. Other useful information provided includes live donation and pediatric transplantation.

The ASTS lists contact information for all of these programs. I reached out to many well before applications were due. Information about individual programs available on their websites varied greatly—some had curriculum and training program goals listed, others merely mentioned that a transplant fellowship existed at the institution. Nearly every program responded, none appeared put off by the contact, and I even received several calls from program directors. It was a great way to learn more about the program prior to applying, and these communications gave me better insight into what programs were looking for in their fellows.

The Interview

The timing of interview offers varies significantly. Many programs will contact you shortly after your application is submitted. Do not worry if you don't receive an offer in short order—some programs have specific days set in advance for interviews and wait until they have reviewed all the applicants before contacting interviewees. Others may contact you to find a day that works for both you and the attendings. I found that most programs were very flexible in working to find a date that worked with my schedule—they understand that you have responsibilities in your residency.

Many programs will have a dinner either the night before or the night of the interview. Try to attend, but I did not find that missing this event precluded me from consideration. Interviews take time, and discussing the time commitments with whoever makes your schedule, your attendings, and your co-residents is essential to having a survivable interview season. My scheduling chief was great about finding solutions to time off requests, and my co-residents made it possible by picking up the slack. It may involve you trading calls or other people covering your responsibilities. The key is early, clear communication with everyone involved. You may end up covering weekend or holiday shifts to get a Wednesday off, but it is a small price to pay. Make sure you aren't violating any of the rules governing your residency, travel on post-call days, and do not let your performance slip. Everyone at your residency wants you to succeed-don't give them a reason to regret their sacrifices.

You must do your homework. Know the history of the program you are visiting. They will generally provide an itinerary for your day, consisting of multiple 30–60-min interviews with transplant attendings and often with nephrology and hepatology physicians. You may also interview with staff such as coordinators, physician assistants, and nurse practitioners. All of the attendings will have CVs available—know where they trained as well as their clinical and research interests. The interviews were not pimping sessions. The attending and staff will be working with you for 2 years; they want to know about your interest in transplant, any focus you may have, what experience you have, but most importantly if you will be a valuable member of the transplant team.

This is your opportunity to learn more about their program—where have recent fellows gone on to practice, how are the responsibilities on the floor and in the clinic handled, who is doing donor operations and what is your involvement, how much research have recent fellows published, and what they expect of you during your training. You may ask about other training you will receive—does the transplant service cover vascular access? Will you be covering hepatic and pancreatic resections for cancer or is that under the surgical oncology team? How involved will you be in living donor and pediatric cases? Common questions I encountered as an interviewee were about the organization of my residency (they want to know if you can be appropriately independent), most common cases I had logged, how I interact in a team and in leadership roles, and how I envision my practice in the future. Be honest and be yourself—better to discover the fit isn't ideal during the interview than 6 months into your training.

You may have the opportunity to participate in rounds or in listing meetings for potential recipients. I found this very valuable, as you experience how the transplant team functions. You will witness how the different specialties interact, who is taking the lead depending on the issue, and how the service runs. Who manages medical issues on a liver recipient 6 months post-op? How about at 1 year? Is renal transplant immunosupression managed by the surgeons or transplant nephrology? Is the fellow running rounds and how involved are the residents? These experiences allow you a glimpse into your future.

Please talk to the fellows. They will likely have moved on to a new hospital (unless they stay on as an attending) before you start, and I found them to be honest, forthright, and generally exhausted. People may caution you about programs that "hide fellows" at interviews, but I did not find this to be an issue. I was always provided contact information, and the fellows I reached out to were willing to talk by phone. They are exhausted for a reason—they are either working or recovering from working. You want to be at a busy program with a ton of operative experience. It is important to get their perspective on their role on the team, the teaching style at the program, and their overall lifestyle. On donor operations, is it an attending walking a fellow through the case, or is it the senior fellow teaching the junior? What is the process to be certified to perform these procedures independently? What cases are they logging and what is the volume? Are cases being double scrubbed by attendings on a frequent basis, and what sorts of cases are double scrubbed? What cases are residents covering with the attending versus with the fellow? How is the food (do not underestimate the importance of this)? Do you know where your call room is?

I found that about half of the programs conducted group interviews and half individual. Group interviews are a great way to get to know your future colleagues—again it's a small world, you will be seeing these people in the future, likely a week later at your next interview. It was a great way to learn what other candidates valued in their education, what their experiences were and their goals. Yes, you are all in competition, but be personable and professional—these interactions are definitely noticed by the staff and administrative assistants who are organizing a day, and they have a voice in selection. Individual interviews are more personal, but you will often have a lot of down time. Make and review notes, bring articles for your upcoming journal club, and get to know the staff. If you look half asleep on your tenth interview of the day, it will leave a bad impression and override the first nine during which you were very engaged.

Ranking

Your rank list will be due in late May. Take a deep breath and don't worry. For positions starting in 2017, 96% of graduates of US residency programs matched—there were 74 active positions and 69% filled. You should keep a running list of the programs you preferred, but it can be difficult to remember every detail after seeing many centers. I put together a spreadsheet that included information that I found to be important to my selection, such as certificates offered, additional training available, live donor transplantation, volume of each case over the past year, etc. I calculated a rough "cases per fellow" number as well. For instance, if a program performed 100 liver transplants per year and took 1 fellow per year, the "cases per fellow" was 50. Yes this is inexact, and most programs have a focus on liver the second year, but you get the idea. A program performing 100 cases a year but taking 2 fellows yearly would be 100/4 current fellows = 25. A program doing 70 livers yearly but taking 1 fellow every other year may allow you to perform more total transplants than a seemingly busier center with many fellows. The NRMP offers an application you can download on your phone that will import the information from the programs you select with a customizable list of center characteristics that can help you organize your priorities and your rank list.

I found that programs fit into three basic categories. "Academic" programs had a strong research component to their curriculum but may offer a lower volume of cases. "Workhorse" programs were very high volume; any research performed was a bonus and discussions about covering clinic were met with snickering—"If you have time, but don't count on it." Finally, there were lower volume programs that offered great training, fewer attendings, and potentially a less chaotic experience.

Only you can decide what experience will best aid you in becoming an outstanding transplant surgeon. Talk to your transplant attendings as they may be able to offer additional insight or answer specific questions you have about a program. Stay in contact with the programs you interviewed with. Obviously you should not mention ranking but it doesn't hurt to remind everyone you enjoyed your visit.

I hope this brief overview answered your questions about the transplant fellowship application process. While stressful, I enjoyed my experience and wish you luck as you enter this amazing field.

Resources

American Society of Transplant Surgeons. http://www.asts.org
The Organ Procurement and Transplantation Network. http://www.optn.transplant.hrsa.gov/data/
The Scientific Registry of Transplant Recipients. http://www.srtr.org

Part II
How to Find a Job

Chapter 12
Where to Look for a Job After Residency

Jonathan Nguyen and Thomas J. Cartolano

Introduction

You've made it! You have spent the better half of your young professional life study-ing, taking tests, staying up all night on call, and missing big events to become a surgeon. Now is the first time you're in high demand, and you're not competing against hundreds of other people for two positions. The mentality of "I can suffer anywhere for 5 (plus) years" no longer applies. Before you start searching for your dream job, decide whether you want an academic or community position and what geographic areas you are comfortable working in. Now start looking for that job using specialty websites, headhunters, locums, and word of mouth. Remember to use some sort of organization system to remember whom you've contacted and fol-low up with them if you really want that position.

What Kind of Job Do I want?

Where do you start your search? Some time and thought must be taken to answer a few critical questions. First, what geographical location do I want to work in? It can be as broad as Northeast, West Coast, and South to more specific areas like New

J. Nguyen, DO (✉)
Division of Trauma and Critical Care, Department of Surgery, Morehouse School of Medicine, Atlanta, GA, USA
e-mail: jnguyen@msm.edu

T. J. Cartolano, DO
Trauma Surgery and Surgical Critical Care, Advocate Christ Medical Center, Oak Lawn, IL, USA

University of Illinois, Chicago, IL, USA

© Springer International Publishing AG, part of Springer Nature 2018
K. Yoon-Flannery et al. (eds.), *A Surgeon's Path*,
https://doi.org/10.1007/978-3-319-78846-3_12

England, Oklahoma, or San Diego. Secondly, what kind of a practice do I want? Academic, private practice, hospital-based practice, or rural surgery?

Academic positions come in a variety of flavors. They all are associated with a university but can vary widely in affiliation. If you choose this route, you have to determine the level of involvement you want. Please see Chap. 20 for more details.

Private practices also vary from a very robust practice in a city to a rural surgical practice. You can work as an employee in a practice with no advancement possibility in sight or work to become a partner (in which case ask what the requirements are to become partner and what it'll cost you). Similarly, some hospitals in smaller communities can offer you hospital employment or bring you in as a private practitioner but supplement your salary for the first few years. Working in these settings can be financially rewarding, and it may involve more benefits including student loan repayment and relocation stipend.

Where Do I Find Jobs?

By understanding where you want to work and what type of practice, you now have a general idea of the kind of position you are looking for, and you can use a few resources to start finding that dream job.

1. Specialty Website—Every specialty has a website that usually contains a list of job openings. This is a great resource to start your search and have access to job openings. For example, trauma has resources such as www.EAST.org and www. AAST.org that list several open positions around the country. The benefit of these websites is that they're free, they have no particular bias, and many institutions around the country use them. The downside is that they may not be up to date and do not represent all possible positions available.

2. Headhunters—These people make their living on finding you a spot. They have a wide network of contacts and can find you a position anywhere across the country. The downside is that while it costs you nothing to use them, the employer usually pays a finder's fee to use their service. That fee can sometimes come at the cost of your signing bonus or some other potential benefit package. And since they get paid on matching you to a job, they don't always have your best interest at heart. "Well I know you wanted that job in 'major metropolitan city,' so I found you a job in 'small town.' It's only 90 min away!" This isn't meant to discourage using them but to be cognizant of what they have to offer and how they operate.

3. Locum Companies—There are several companies who specialize in placing you in desirable positions for a short period of time. The benefit here is that the work pays well, they take care of the travel and lodging expenses, and can help you buy time as you wait for a significant other, or find the job you really want. You

should, however, keep in mind that it is temporary work and you may be moving on to a new place in only a few months. Furthermore, benefits are not always included.

4. Word of Mouth—This is self-explanatory, but you'd be surprised who knows whom. Ask your attendings, mentors, and any other connections you have developed over the years to put in a good word for you.

Final Words

As you start applying for these positions, keep a spreadsheet of the institutions and contact information including phone numbers and e-mail addresses. Check in from time to time if you haven't heard back for a while. Keep an open mind and talk with your mentors to get an idea of what is really important to you. Don't be discouraged if your *dream job* doesn't reveal itself right away. The position that was a hard *no* on your list may turn out to be a high contender, and that dream job may turn out to be a bust. At the end of the day, don't panic because this decision doesn't have to be the only job you take. If the position doesn't mesh with your style, you can always look somewhere else.

Just remember, 50% of physicians end up switching jobs in the first 2 years. There are plenty of people in the same boat as you, and people move on.

Chapter 13
Job Applications

Rose E. Mustafa and Jonathan Nguyen

Introduction

You have (almost) made it! You have finally completed training, either in general surgery or your fellowship (or close to it). Congratulations!! *You did it*!! It is a big deal. Celebrate. Have a glass of wine, or three. Sleep in. Wake up. Take a deep breath, and let us begin again.

After selling yourself to programs for the past 5–10 years of your life, you will be pleasantly surprised to see that the hospitals, medical centers, and institutions are finally being sold TO YOU. This chapter will provide some perspectives on how to organize and manage this next big step.

Preparation

Employment opportunities will arise from all different angles. Be ready. Have your CV and cover letter ready to email within seconds if prompted. Your impressive CV is full of your accomplishments to date. Fine-tune it. Have your mentors and/or program directors give you feedback on your final CV. Also, remember to update your CV as the year goes along. If you are in your fellowship year, you are likely still producing research, writing chapters, and completing assignments, and this should all be reflected in your CV.

R. E. Mustafa, MD (✉)
Breast Surgical Oncologist, Saint Peter's University Hospital,
Saint Peter's Breast Center, New Brunswick, NJ, USA

J. Nguyen, DO
Division of Trauma and Critical Care, Department of Surgery, Morehouse School
of Medicine, Atlanta, GA, USA

© Springer International Publishing AG, part of Springer Nature 2018
K. Yoon-Flannery et al. (eds.), *A Surgeon's Path*,
https://doi.org/10.1007/978-3-319-78846-3_13

Cover Letters

Cover letters should provide a concise summary of who you are, what type of practice you would thrive in, what you are looking for, and what you have to offer. Personalize each cover letter to the institution of interest, and send it along with your CV.

CVs and Resumes

What's the difference? We feel like the terms are all interchangeable, and the template we used in high school should still work for this position. Unfortunately, that is incorrect. The major difference is that a CV trims the fat. Your parents are still proud that you had perfect attendance throughout your junior high career, but no one else is. Remove the things that don't add significance to your CV. Keep the things that are pertinent to you as a surgeon, mentor, administrator, educator, researcher, and leader. Make sure the font matches and that the format is consistent. Remember, as surgeons, we don't like to waste time. Make sure your CV flows well and conveys your surgical prowess. Ensure the contact information is up to date. It is never a bad idea to ask a senior resident, fellow, program director, or mentor to review your CV once you have compiled it. Many times this person can look at the big picture and give you very helpful feedback. Bottom line is that you don't want to be the only person who has looked at your CV besides the people you are sending it to.

Application

After you have figured out where in the country you would like to begin this next chapter, start applying! There are job boards through national societies and recruiters who will inevitably contact you by phone, text, email, and snail mail. Program directors usually are notified of open positions prior to opportunities being publicly posted, so make sure you are in constant communication with them. Word of mouth goes a long way. Contact your previous chiefs and co-residents that are in the field or geographical location you are interested in. Ask if there are unpublicized opportunities arising and have them put in a good word. As we have previously stated in this book, the world of surgery is a lot smaller than you think. Someone always knows someone, who trained with someone else, who happens to know the chief of surgery of the hospital you are applying to. Use this to your benefit. It is NOT uncommon for graduating residents/fellows to contact previous mentors, attendings, or colleagues that they haven't spoken to in years for any potential professional opportunities. Applications are submitted in different formats for every opportunity. They can be submitted via the hospital websites, direct contact with recruiters, department assistants, or via email. There is always *Room for error*. Make sure you *follow up*. Confirm the receipt of your CV and cover letter in the proper hands.

The application and interview process takes weeks to months; therefore it is imperative that you begin to apply early. Many times this can be at the beginning of an academic year for a job you will not start until July or August. During the year, you may attend national meetings or networking events, where you will meet individuals who would potentially play a major role in your future. This is an opportunity for you to disclose your interest and allow them to put a face to the name on the CV. During these opportunities, ask your attendings and mentors to introduce you to people they know. If it doesn't help this time around, it may the next.

There are usually multiple interviews scheduled weeks apart. The process can be different for every institution, but you can expect to start with a phone interview followed by an on-site first interview, and if both parties are interested in pursuing a professional relationship, most of the time, you are called back for a second interview.

A term sheet is generally provided at this point which is usually a one-page summary including important information such as:

Contract term (usually first agreements are 1–3 year contracts).
Compensation.
Benefits including relocation reimbursement, pension, vacation, and CME allowance.
Noncompete clause.
Refer to the *Contracts and Negotiations* chapter 15 for more information on this.

Communication

Communicate with your current program. Ensure that your program director, the attending you are working with, and your rotating surgical team are ALL aware of upcoming interviews. Attempt to schedule interviews on days where there may be least disruption to the team you are currently on, but keep in mind that interviewing for jobs is just as important as other duties of your residency or fellowship. Your future job will reflect your current program, and they should be supportive of your application and interviews. Follow up and make sure the mentors you solicited for letters and paperwork complete and send out those important documents. Offer to help to ensure these things get done in a timely manner.

Narrow Down Your Choices

At this point in your career, you likely have a system in place as to how you make important decisions. Some colleagues have used EXCEL sheets to place all the information and use a point system to decide. Some people have highly respected mentors that have led them to success thus far and trust their opinion. Some colleagues say that "it just felt right," and that's that. So, to each their own!

Consider your options. Salary is important. People say it isn't, but it is. You have student loans that have accrued tons of interest, and you have run out of forbearance and deferment options. Keep in mind, however, salary as a single number can be deceiving. As noted above, there are multiple ways in which you can be appropriately compensated. Areas where this can be particularly unique among positions include CME allowance, retirement or tuition benefits, bonus structure, and administrative and clinical support staff.

So yes. Salary is important, but so is your happiness. Advice that has been consistently shared with us is make sure you can work with your new colleagues. The personality, work ethic, and even humor of your co-workers could make for a wonderfully successful and supportive early career or a miserably malignant slow tread through the first few years of early attending-hood. Get a feel for how the current staff get along. Do they support each other and have fun? Do they barely make eye contact? See if there is a mentor within them also. Who will help you navigate the new system and watch your back? Who will help you succeed and prevent you from getting into trouble?

A mentor along the way once said, "I want to hire someone that I can be with at 3 o' clock in the morning. If nothing is going on, they are someone I can shoot the shit with, but they are also the ones I want to stand next to when all hell is breaking loose."

Final Words

This is an exciting time in which you are now being highly sought after. Enjoy the moment and then prepare for the next phase. Prepare by identifying those who will support and back you with phone calls and letters. Polish your CV, cover letters, and letters of recommendation. Systematically apply for the programs in the regions and practices you want, and follow up with them. Don't be afraid to be persistent. When you start interviewing, make sure that the position posted is actually what's being offered and that it jives with what you want.

Chapter 14
Interviewing for Your First Job

Asanthi M. Ratnasekera

Introduction

The interview process is your first opportunity to show up and make an impression on your future employer. This is also your opportunity to familiarize yourself with your prospective employer, hospital, staff, director, and future partners. Although you may be only seeing a glimpse of what happens in daily life at this certain practice or hospital, you can at least get an idea of how things look on the surface.

Preparation for Interview

Prior to your interview, it is important to understand the demographics of your future hospital or practice. It is important to know if the location is where you would want to practice as a physician for the next 3–5 years of your life. Understand that this may not be your one and only job for the rest of your life. Statistics have shown that many people leave their first job as an attending for a greater opportunity.

If you have already applied for a job and received an interview, adequate research on the institution or practice must be done ahead of time. Here are some recommendations for things to consider when researching this job:

1. Is this the type of institution you wish to practice in? For example, you need to consider academic vs. nonacademic, large, or small community hospitals and private practice or hospital-based employment.
2. What is the presence of surgical residents and midlevel providers that are there for support of the team?

A. M. Ratnasekera, DO
Crozer-Keystone Health System, Upland, PA, USA

© Springer International Publishing AG, part of Springer Nature 2018
K. Yoon-Flannery et al. (eds.), *A Surgeon's Path*,
https://doi.org/10.1007/978-3-319-78846-3_14

As with many aspects of your career, it is helpful to have mentorship and guidance to answer these questions. You may have a strong idea that you want to end up in academics or you may be unsure about the difference between private practice and hospital-based employment. It is important to ask people that you trust about making these choices. These are *not* the questions you should be asking on interview day.

Make travel plans early. Most practices or hospital systems will accommodate travel and lodging for your interview. The administrative assistant should assist you in making plans for your travel arrangements. Most interviews will take place during the day, and some places will offer a dinner with your future partners and/or director prior to the day of the interview. This is the time to observe the dynamics between partners and their behaviors in a casual setting.

The next step is to research the faculty and future partners and the director.

1. Are they from an academic background that would give you adequate mentorship especially in your first job?
2. What are their research interests if any and do they match yours?

Even though on paper everything may look bright and shiny, the surgical community is a small world and people know each other. It is nice to ask around about partners and directors to get a global idea of people's reputations.

Interview Day

Interview day is not only an opportunity to showcase your professionalism and your resume but also to be observant of the practice, hospital environment, and your (potential) future partners. Always arrive to your interview a few minutes early. Give yourself time to battle traffic, to find the location of the interview, and to park. Obviously professional attire is a must. Interview day is the short window you have for observing the hospital flow, how easy is it to get from one place to another, where the clinic, office, call rooms, and operating rooms are located. This is also an excellent opportunity to meet with the junior partners and ask them about their experience. Some suggested questions for your interview day include:

1. Has there been adequate support and mentoring for junior faculty career advancement?
2. Are the partners available in case you need help?
3. What type of call schedule can you expect?
4. What kind of nursing and midlevel support can you expect early in practice or within a couple of years?

Follow-Up

A second interview may or may not be offered. It is probably helpful to ask about this at the end of your first interview so you have an idea of what to expect. It's always courteous to thank the director for the opportunity to interview and to express your level of interest in that institution. If you have found another opportunity in the meantime, it is respectful to inform the institutions about your unavailability to pursue this job offer further.

Chapter 15
Contract Negotiation

Kahyun Yoon-Flannery and Jonathan Nguyen

Introduction

Starting the interview trail for your first position after training can be quite a daunting process. It can involve traveling to far and unfamiliar places, meeting new people, and trying to figure out whether your potential new partners and new employer are a good fit for you or not. Of course, you also want to impress the people you are meeting. We are surgeons after all, perfectionists bred from the beginning, and hearing "no" as an answer certainly is undesirable and unacceptable. So after multiple rounds of what feels like an awkward first date, you are ready to see what they have to offer. We certainly did not have any preexisting knowledge of what a fair employment contract should look like but along the way acquired some knowledge. Here are some pearls of wisdom that we have passed down to our colleagues and friends.

Finding a Physician Contract Attorney

If there is one thing you can take away from this chapter, it is that you absolutely need to seek legal counsel before even coming *close* to signing your first contract. And you really want an experienced contract attorney who is not only familiar with physician specific contracts but is specialty specific as well. One of our partners is actually an attorney, and at the beginning, we honestly thought that he could take a quick look at whatever offers we received and we could save some money. He is a land use and zoning attorney with no experience in these sorts of contracts. When

K. Yoon-Flannery, DO, MPH (✉)
Sidney Kimmel Cancer Center, Jefferson Health New Jersey, Sewell, NJ, USA
e-mail: kahyun.yoon-flannery@jefferson.edu

J. Nguyen, DO
Division of Trauma and Critical Care, Morehouse School of Medicine, Atlanta, GA, USA

© Springer International Publishing AG, part of Springer Nature 2018
K. Yoon-Flannery et al. (eds.), *A Surgeon's Path*,
https://doi.org/10.1007/978-3-319-78846-3_15

we questioned as to why we needed to spend extra money on legal counsel, his response was "that request is the equivalent of me asking you to do orthopedic surgery on me." Point taken. You also want to seek counsel from someone who comes recommended to you by those who actually experienced their services firsthand. Our attorney was recommended by multiple different physician mentors whom we trusted implicitly, and in return we recommended his services to many of our resident and fellowship friends after our experiences.

The amount of legal fees one is expected to spend can be widely ranging depending on where you are located and to what extent you need legal services. An attorney can offer a flat fee for service or offer an hourly rate. From what we had researched (mostly through word of mouth), the range we saw in the Philadelphia region, where one of us currently practice, was anywhere from $500 to $3000. There were some services offered through physician organizations that offered a nominal flat fee, but the big caveat was that you did not find out who your attorney was until AFTER you made a payment. Our advice to you is that you should certainly research which attorney and which law firm are widely used for your specific field of specialty. And don't worry too much about what they are charging you. This is certainly one of the most important investments you NEED to make at the beginning of your career. After all was done, we wholeheartedly believe that our attorney's advice was worth MUCH more than what he charged us (but don't tell him that).

Salary

Salary is certainly one of the foremost things on your mind. How one comes up with what is an appropriate level of salary for your level of expertise and locale is somewhat of a mystery. There are some resources, however, that will help you become aware of "what you are worth" generally. One of the most important resources is the annual salary data published from the Medical Group Management Association (MGMA). MGMA releases average salary information based on level of experience and location and breaks down salary based on specialties. Every employer we encountered quoted or made a comparison to what had been published in MGMA. You can purchase a copy of the data from their website, http://www.mgma.com, or obtain the data from other sources. An experienced physician contract attorney will have the most recent data and will be able to provide it to you so you have a reference. The only caveat is that this data is solely based on physician surveys, and some categories do not have a high level of participation for their surveys. So it may not be entirely accurate regarding the current rate in your area, but it is certainly a great starting point, and you should arm yourself with this information.

The best way to gauge what you are worth is by asking your colleagues. Now this can be a sensitive topic since certainly discussing one's salary is a very private subject, and not everyone will be forthcoming. Fortunately, we had a number of mentors who were very frank about what they had been offered and what their trajectory for increase in salary was. This takes some effort, and you must rely on some of the personal relationships you have developed along the way, but we found it to be one of the most important tools to have through this process. Many contracts will stipulate, however, that you are not legally allowed to discuss the details of your contract with those other than your attorney or your family members. So you should certainly read the fine print when giving out advice.

When discussing your salary, you also want to think about how your time is parsed out especially if you have responsibilities for administrative work, research, or education. The term full-time employee (FTE) is often used and in theory determines how much of your time is dedicated to clinical work. Make sure your percentages are adding up to no more than 100%.

Bonus Structure

Every contract can be personalized to a certain extent. A lot of the surgeon contracts will include some sort of bonus structure, and it will likely be based on work relative value units (wRVUs). Basically, every procedure or patient visit you have as a physician will have some sort of a set wRVU associated with it, and you can usually gauge what is supposed to be an average yearly wRVU total based on your specialty and the location in which you practice. And a bonus structure will usually include either a fee per wRVU beyond the agreed yearly average total wRVU or a flat bonus fee based on a number of agreed quality metrics measures on a yearly basis. You want to be aware of what is a reasonable amount of wRVUs, based on your specialty and your level of training, and also what type of a practice you are joining. It usually will take a minimum of 1–2 years of ramping up for you to have a fully functioning practice, and thus agreeing to an "average" amount of wRVUs in the beginning of your career, and your contract period may not be a reasonable option for you. Also, your specialty may affect your wRVU output. For example, what is expected for you as a bariatric surgeon in a robust practice with an existing referral pattern may be entirely different from what one would expect to produce as a breast surgeon. The wRVU data are also available through MGMA and certainly should be obtained prior to your making specific negotiation points. And do not be afraid to ask your mentors what their average annual wRVUs are.

In addition, you may want to inquire about a sign-on bonus, especially if you are joining a practice that is in dire need of a specialist in your area of expertise with your level of training. The amount of the sign-on bonus can certainly have a wide range, and the terms by which it is paid can also vary. In our experience, a sign-on bonus usually has some kind of a payment schedule where you receive a portion at the time of signing of the contract, with the remainder of the bonus being parsed out through multiple time periods during your employment period. You can also expect to see a "retention bonus," where after completing your first year of practice and having maintained all agreed contract points, you receive a lump sum. Again, speaking with your colleagues in your general practice area and specialty will be invaluable to determine what bonuses you may receive. Alternatively, some organizations give out bonuses under the guise of a "loan" from the hospital, provided that you honor "X" numbers of years with them and meet their contract points. In this situation, if you fail to do so, you owe the hospital the entire "loan" plus interest, in whole, at that time.

Malpractice Insurance

You certainly want the specifics of malpractice coverage spelled out in your contract. There are two types of malpractice insurance: "claims-made" and "occurrence" coverage. Occurrence coverage protects you for the rest of your life for any claim that happens during the time of the policy. Claims-made coverage protects you from claims happening during the time of the policy that is also filed during the time of the policy. You work at the hospital from 2008 to 2010. If you're sued in 2010 about an event that happened in 2009, both policies cover you. If you're sued in 2012 about an event that happened in 2009, only the occurrence based coverage will protect you. In this case you want malpractice coverage not only for cases that may occur during your employment period but also for cases that may develop after you have left your employer, i.e., "tail coverage." Usually your employer will want to specify that you must be able to obtain the required insurance for the employer to honor this clause (i.e., the employer doesn't want to pay an exorbitant amount of malpractice coverage because you already have so many outstanding cases against you). Our recommendation is that you specify that the coverage be obtained at "standard reasonable rates within your specialty for malpractice insurance coverage."

Benefits

There are several components under the Benefits section of the contract that require your attention. You want to negotiate the maximum amount of vacation, sick, and holiday time you are entitled to on a yearly basis. In addition, you also want to ensure that there are provisions for Continuing Medical Education (CME) courses, as well as for maintaining your licensure. What we have found is that while there is a wide range, you should see at least $5000–$7500 on a yearly basis to cover your CME courses and your licensure. You may also be entitled to a separate number of days allotted for CME courses. During our contract negotiation, we found that 5 days are typically the standard for physician contracts, unless your role is as a department head or equivalent. In addition, you may want to inquire about other benefits such as relocation reimbursement and student loan repayment. From an employer standpoint, a student loan repayment can be a tax write-off, so it may be a more attractive secondary benefit for them to offer you than other benefits. To some degree this benefits section is just as important as the salary, (if not more important). It certainly can be the more flexible component of your contract to negotiate.

Another form of benefits you want to discuss is for maternity/paternity leave. The United States is one of the very few developed countries in the world that still does not guarantee federally mandated paid family leave. New Jersey and California currently do offer state-based benefits, but the amount of paperwork involved and the amount of benefits you actually end up getting will certainly not be enough, even if you happen to practice in one of those states. If you have not yet completed your family, you certainly should discuss the details of a maternity/paternity leave in terms of duration and amount of benefits.

Noncompete Clause

This clause is very important. It is estimated that at least 50% of physicians will leave their first employer after their first contract term is carried out. That means you want to think about where you would be able to practice if things did not work out for you. As you are starting out in your first position, you may be starting a young family as well, and moving your family especially if children are involved may not be an easy task. We once heard from a colleague in a major metropolitan area whose noncompete clause stated that if he ever left the practice, he would not be able to practice anywhere within a 50-mile radius. That means if he ever wanted to leave his existing practice, he would have to uproot his family to an entirely different metro area. The noncompete clause will specify the distance as well as the time period during which you will not be allowed to practice nearby. You may actually want to map out the nearby hospitals or practices and calculate the distances before signing off on this clause.

Miscellaneous

There are other important aspects of your contract that you certainly need to think about as a surgeon, including staffing, call coverage, call schedule (if multiple partners), and OR block time. Depending on what type of a practice you are joining, chances are the practice already has an existing set of support staff dedicated to current physician partners. You want to make sure that you have ample staff members who are dedicated to you. We have a friend who was verbally promised a robust staff, but when she ultimately started, she was informed that she was sharing a single medical assistant with two other partners and that no other nurses or nurse practitioners would be available for her practice for the unforeseeable future. Call coverage or schedule is certainly something you want to include as well. When one of us was entertaining multiple contracts, some contracts actually included a clause where we would be required to cover general surgery emergency room calls, which was unacceptable to us (One of us is a fellowship trained breast surgeon). Lastly, OR block time and your schedule structure in general are also important things for you to discuss in detail prior to signing your contract. Certainly you may need some ramp-up time to build your practice, and you may not be booking actual cases for several months as a practicing surgeon. Nonetheless, you want to have some sense of when your operative days and office days will be, rather than completely having to rely on an "add-on" schedule. As a breast surgeon, "adding on" cancer surgeries just was not feasible, and we certainly discussed all these in details in *writing*, prior to finalizing our contract.

Marketing is another component you want your employer to discuss. Most surgeons will have to rely on a referral pattern, and therefore as a new physician on the block, marketing you and your program will be important.

Final Thoughts

In general, you should be entertaining more than one contract offer before making a final decision. You should never feel rushed to make a decision. One place we interviewed asked me to "make a commitment" on our second interview without showing us any contract whatsoever. We declined to make any kind of verbal agreement and asked to see a detailed contract from them. Upon reviewing, we found it to be a terrible contract that was very pro-employer. You should be able to spend time reviewing various points of your contract, with the help of legal counsel, and the employers should make every effort to allow you to do so.

At the end of the day, however, only you know what would make you happy. There are so many circumstances by which one makes a final commitment to a job. You may not have a lot of flexibility in terms of where you can practice, based on your current family situation. You may already be well-off where a base salary may not mean that much to you, and you would rather have ample vacation time every year. Only you can decide what is a reasonable offer you are willing to accept. And, of course, every contract has an end date if things ultimately do not work out for the best.

Chapter 16
Gender Inequality in Compensation in Medicine and Surgery

Kahyun Yoon-Flannery

My co-chief Mohamed and I started our surgery rotation together as interns. We would make rounds together, where all the beautiful nurses would fawn over him, calling him "Oh, Dr. Mohamed" asking if he needed any help at all. "Oh you need a gauze?" The ladies would run out to the supply closet at the drop of a hat. In the meantime, I'm making rounds with my coat pockets filled with every imaginable supply known to man. I talk to every patient and explain why they have to go to surgery, obtain informed consent, and then go back to check on them when they come out of the operating room. After a few days of taking care of the same patient, he asks me: "Can you bring me oatmeal tomorrow? I really don't like grits. And is my doctor going to ever come and see me?"

To say I was vocal during my general surgery residency training is probably an understatement. I was heavily involved in the contract renegotiation process for all the residents in the university hospital I belonged to and spent countless meetings in the middle of the night arguing with the seasoned labor law attorneys sitting on the other side of the table. When the time came to decide on the topic of my grand rounds presentation as a chief surgical resident, I had just finished the book *Lean In*, by Sheryl Sandberg. This book opened my eyes. Yes, I had always been a vocal female physician, but this book let me evaluate our society as a whole and in a systematic way. So I decided to dedicate my grand rounds talk to discuss gender inequality in medicine and surgery. My talk lasted 1 hour and was attended by many residents, medical students, as well as attending surgeons. It generated a lot of questions, some very thoughtful and some very skeptical at best. But it opened some doors for these types of discussion in a department where for many years talking about "gender" and "female surgeons" was tolerated at best.

The reason I became a physician was possibly to spite my teachers in kindergarten. It is still fresh in my mind; one day we were all asked to play dress-up for what we

K. Yoon-Flannery, DO, MPH
Sidney Kimmel Cancer Center, Jefferson Health New Jersey, Sewell, NJ, USA
e-mail: kahyun.yoon-flannery@jefferson.edu

© Springer International Publishing AG, part of Springer Nature 2018   81
K. Yoon-Flannery et al. (eds.), *A Surgeon's Path*,
https://doi.org/10.1007/978-3-319-78846-3_16

Fig. 16.1 Humorous photo showing gender stereotypes in medicine. (Courtesy of @ doctordconline on Instagram)

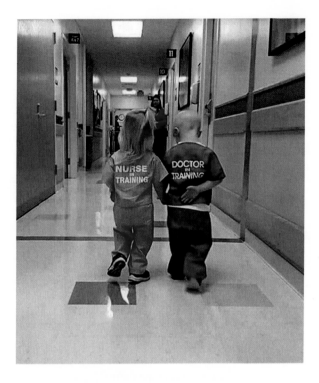

wanted to be when we grew up. I went to the "medical station," 5 years old and very proud, and tried to grab a stethoscope. "Oh no," my teacher said, "You want to wear this." She handed me a nurse's cap. I threw it down in defiance and got in trouble. That was the day I decided I was going to become a doctor and show the world (Fig. 16.1).

The earliest account of women in surgery dates back to 3500 BC at the banks of the Tigris and Euphrates rivers in Mesopotamia [1]. In ancient Greece, Aesculapius, son of Apollo, had four daughters who were all physicians. But as history would have it, women were slowly actively discouraged from having roles in surgery, particularly in the Middle Ages. In 1313, women were banned from practicing surgery in Paris unless they were examined by a "competent" jury. King Henry VIII made a famous declaration in the fourteenth century: "No carpenter, smith, weaver, or women shall practice surgery."

Dr. Elizabeth Blackwell was the first female physician in the United States [2]. She was allowed admission to Geneva Medical College, which is now SUNY Upstate Medical University, after being rejected from more than 20 medical schools. She was only admitted to Geneva after a poll was taken by her colleagues who voted to have her admitted as their classmate. She graduated in 1849 with a gold medal and eventually started and oversaw the Women's Medical College of New York from 1862 to 1899. In honor of Dr. Blackwell's achievements, February 3, her birthday, is now celebrated as the National Women Physician day. The first female surgeon in the United States was Dr. Mary Edwards Walker [3]. She was the second

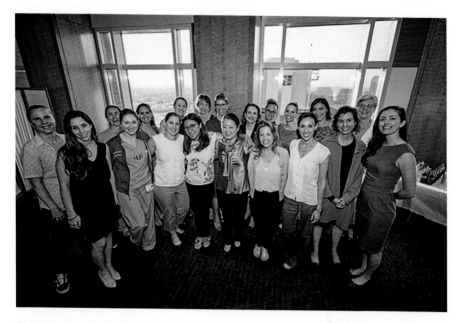

Fig. 16.2 May 26, 2017 Women in Surgery event at the University of Pennsylvania. (Photo by Ed Cunicelli)

female graduate of an American medical school in 1855 from Syracuse Medical College and the first female surgeon in the US Army. She received the Congressional Medal of Honor in 1865.

Women made up about 5% of all physicians in the United States in 1970, but this number rose to 24% in 2001. A 2016 Association of American Medical Colleges (AAMC) report estimated that new enrollment in medical school in 2016 was evenly divided between women (49.8%) and men (50.2%) [4]. As we climb up the ladder, however, the divide becomes greater between men and women in medicine. Women only make up 38% of full-time academic faculty, 21% of full-time professors, 15% of department chairs, and only 16% of medical school deans. In the field of surgery, the proportion of women becomes even smaller, with women representing only 22% of full-time faculty and 1% of department chairs in the United States [5] (Fig. 16.2).

This staggering difference between men and women in medicine becomes perhaps more relevant when we examine compensation data. The Equal Pay Act was only signed into law in 1963 by President Kennedy protecting employees from wage discrimination on the basis of sex. At that time, women earned less than 60% of what men made, which means a female college graduate working full time year round would have made less than the average male high school graduate. Physician compensation data show that although we have made some progress, the pay gap still remains considerable [6–12]. The 2015 Medscape Physician Compensation Report showed that male physicians earn nearly 23% more than female counterparts with an average salary for male physicians of $249,000 as compared to $203,000 for female physicians [10]. A US nationwide survey of recipients of NIH K08 and K23 grants confirmed this gender bias in salary for physicians. The reported mean salary was $167,669 for women compared to $200,433 for men in this study. This study also found that the male gender was associated with higher salary, even after adjusting for specialty, academic rank, leadership positions, publications, and research time.

A 2011 Health Affairs study showed that not only do female physicians earn less, but the discrepancy was getting increasingly worse, growing from an average of $3600 gap in 1999 to a $16,819 differential in 2008 [8]. Another interesting finding from this study was that men initiate negotiations about four times more often than women, and on average, even when women negotiate, they receive 30% less than men [10].

When it was time for me to entertain different contracts for myself, I took these data to heart. I wanted to negotiate to the highest amount for *any* surgeon, male or female. I spoke to every possible person I could think of and sought out their advice in terms of details of their contracts, including salary and other forms of compensation. Knowledge really is power. Knowing what other surgeons in the area were able to command gave me the ability to make more demands.

But here I sit, after having signed the best contract I could ask for, thinking well, what else can I do? What else can we do so that we continue to close the gender gap in medicine and surgery? On both institutional and personal levels, we need to mentor both men *and* women. Yale School of Medicine has established an Office for Women in Medicine whose mission is to promote the growth of women in academic medicine and medical sciences. Wherever we are, we can do our part by providing our physicians, both men and women, access to advisors and mentors, as well as sponsoring lectures by bringing distinguished women in medicine as role models. We can also provide a safe forum where young physicians can come together to discuss their professional development and career opportunities. We also need to be able to have open discussions on salary. Many of the contracts I was given did not allow me to discuss the details of my contract with other physicians. Why? Having knowledge of what others were earning personally was the reason I felt so prepared.

One of the first things we learn as physicians is that we have to treat our patients without prejudice. We have to treat everyone equally regardless of sex, socioeconomic status, insurance status, or religious beliefs. As such, I would hope to be treated by my own patients and colleagues as a surgeon in general regardless of what I may represent from a personalized perspective.

References

1. Wirtzfeld DA. The history of women in surgery. Can J Surg. 2009;52(4):317–20.
2. Sabin F. Elizabeth Blackwell: the first woman doctor. New York: Troll Communications; 1982.

3. Walker DL. Mary Edwards Walker; above and beyond. New York: Tom Doherty Associates; 2005.
4. Lautenberger DM, et al. The state of women in academic medicine: the pipeline and pathways to leadership: Association of American Medical Colleges; 2014. https://members.aamc.org/eweb/upload/The%20State%20of%20Women%20in%20Academic%20Medicine%202013-2014. 20FINAL.pdf
5. Davis EC, et al. Women in surgery residency programs: evolving trends from a national perspective. J Am Coll Surg. 2011;212:320–6.
6. Coontz S. Progress at work, but mothers still pay a price. The New York Times, Sunday Review 2013 Jun 8. http://www.nytimes.com/2013/06/09/opinion/sunday/coontz-richer-childless-women-are-making-the-gains.html?_r=0
7. Jagsi R, et al. Gender differences in the salaries of physician researchers. JAMA. 2012;307(22):2410–7.
8. Lo Sasso AT, et al. The $16,819 pay gap for newly trained physicians: the unexplained trend of men earning more than women. Health Aff. 2011;30(2):193–201.
9. Merrill A. Why are women so underrepresented in surgery leadership? Huffington Post 2015 Sept 10. http://www.huffingtonpost.com/andrea-merrill/women-surgeons_b_8079896.html
10. Reese S. Do women doctors need to negotiate more assertively? Medscape News & Perspective 2015 Aug 05. http://www.medscape.com/viewarticle/848309?src=wnl_edit_bom_weekly&uac=113161EG&impID=788536&faf=1
11. Brodwin E, Nudelman M. Here's how much money doctors actually make. Business Insider 2017 Apr 5. http://www.businessinsider.com/how-much-money-do-doctors-make-2017-4
12. Kowalczyk L. Female surgeons say explicit bias is rare, but subtler obstacles still exist in Boston. Boston Globe 2015 Feb 25. http://archive.boston.com/lifestyle/health/2013/02/25/female-surgeons-say-explicit-bias-rare-but-subtler-obstacles-still-exist-boston/CqDZ25e2R1g8IL4ky4LzKJ/story.html

Suggested Reading

Davis K. 5 practical things men can do for gender equality at work. Fast Company 2014 Oct 21. http://www.fastcompany.com/3037193/strong-female-lead/5-practical-things-men-can-do-for-gender-equality-at-work
Hutchingson AM. Pregnancy and childbirth during family medicine residency training. Fam Med. 2011;43(3):160–5.
Miller NH. Pregnancies among physicians. A historical cohort Study. J Reprod Med. 1989;34:790–6.
Office for Women in Medicine: Yale School of Medicine. http://medicine.yale.edu/owm
Tamburrino MB. Physician pregnancy: male and female colleagues' attitudes. J Am Med Wom Assoc. 1992;48:82–4.
Turner PL. Pregnancy among women surgeons. Arch Surg. 2012;147(5):474–9.

Chapter 17
Applying for Privileges and Licensure

Jonathan Nguyen

Introduction

After completing years of training, you are just a few steps away from starting your career. You've figured out your dream job and are ready to start. The only thing standing in your way is your mortal enemy—paperwork. The unfortunate truth is that paperwork is the ever-pervasive entity in your life, and before starting your job, you'll have to jump through these hoops too.

Licensure

No matter where you plan to practice, you'll need a state license, and you can be sure that the process is slow and painful. Once you've identified the state or states you want to practice in, start the process. Some of the states that have a notoriously long process are Texas, Florida, and California. These states can take well over 6 months to complete the process, and Texas even requires that you take a jurisprudence exam. To find the licensure board, a simple web search for the state and medical license will suffice. Make sure that your information is up to date and that you give a reliable address. There are also medical licensing service firms that will help you through this application process for a fee. Using these services can be helpful since you only fill out the information once, and the service sends all the appropriate data for you.

J. Nguyen, DO
Division of Trauma and Critical Care, Department of Surgery, Morehouse School of Medicine, Atlanta, GA, USA
e-mail: jnguyen@msm.edu

© Springer International Publishing AG, part of Springer Nature 2018
K. Yoon-Flannery et al. (eds.), *A Surgeon's Path*,
https://doi.org/10.1007/978-3-319-78846-3_17

Once you've gotten your state license, you can now apply for your license for the US Drug Enforcement Administration (DEA). The application requires a state license to associate with, and you can apply here at https://apps.deadiversion.usdoj. gov/webforms/. This can take several weeks to months. Usually your employer can reimburse the costs involved with these license applications so you should certainly check your benefits and save all your documentation. If for some reason you cannot use these for reimbursement through your employer, you can try to claim these as part of your deductions on your tax return. Communication with your colleagues and partners along with your administrative support staff will help guide your application process.

Privileges

After you accept your contract, your employer will likely start sending you packets of paperwork to fill out. This includes forms for hospital privileges to care for patients and perform procedures. At some point of your application, you will be asked what procedures you'd like to do. Put down *everything*. It's much easier to take off procedures later than to try to add them and prove you are proficient. They'll ask for someone to corroborate your requests, so make sure to have your program director sign off on them. Prior to the completion of your training, make sure you save a copy of your operative logs from residency and fellowship training. This will be very helpful especially if you're asking for special privileges for uncommon procedures.

Keep scanned copies of your certifications, diplomas, and letters in a clearly labeled file on your computer. You may need to submit these documents to various organizations and employer multiple times, and it will save you time if you keep them organized in an electronic format.

Stay in close contact with your office manager and the hospital credentialing office staff to ensure there are no new items popping up. And if you actually have to send anything via mail, always send it with tracking.

Insurance Enrollment

Once you get the job and finish your paperwork for state license and hospital privileges, there is still more paperwork to complete! Next comes a stack of forms from every insurance provider you'll come in contact with, including Medicare and Medicaid. They all ask the same information, and you'll spend a full day checking boxes and writing down the same information. My experience is that hospital credentialing staff will be providing you with assistance and to keep track of what is still outstanding. All this can take weeks to months to finalize, so it is important to file all paperwork as soon as possible. The last thing you would want is to start working and realize you cannot bill for the services you are providing your patients.

Final Remarks

The process for obtaining your state licensure and privileges is not difficult, but it does take time. Be sure to *start early* and keep organized. If you have an idea of the state(s) you want to practice in, start the paperwork ASAP. You may be able to have the university staff help you prior to your graduation, especially if you are staying within the same state to practice. Finalizing these details as early as possible will certainly be to your advantage as well as your employers.

Chapter 18
Moving

Anuradha Reema Kar and Elliott R. Haut

Introduction

Congratulations! You have matched in fellowship or have gotten the dream job you have been working toward for a decade! Unfortunately, now you have to uproot your entire life and start over in a completely new zip code. Moving is a daunting task, even for people accustomed to high-pressure situations as surgeons. Luckily, you are likely a type A personality who mastered the art of checklists by the second week of internship. Detailed planning is essential to complete as stress-free a move as possible. We provide a simplified framework to follow when planning your relocation, whether you are moving across the country or down the street.

What Is the Big Picture?

Invest in a large paper calendar (or computerized equivalent) and mark out the important dates. Start as early as possible! Unfortunately, graduating surgery residents are not the only people moving in the middle of summer. The rest of the world likes moving during the warmer months, too. This makes spring and summer a competitive season for finding housing and arranging commercial movers. The sooner you start planning, the more likely you will be able to find the most cost-effective

A. R. Kar, MD (✉)
Acute Care Surgery, Trauma, Burns and Critical Care, Department of Surgery,
Johns Hopkins University School of Medicine, Baltimore, MD, USA
e-mail: reemakar@jhmi.edu

E. R. Haut, MD, PhD, FACS
Division of Trauma Surgery and Critical Care, Department of Surgery,
Johns Hopkins University School of Medicine, Baltimore, MD, USA
e-mail: ehaut1@jhmi.edu

© Springer International Publishing AG, part of Springer Nature 2018
K. Yoon-Flannery et al. (eds.), *A Surgeon's Path*,
https://doi.org/10.1007/978-3-319-78846-3_18

and time-efficient moving schedule, especially if you have a narrow window in which to relocate.

Once you have outlined the broad dates, focus on the specifics. When is the last day you can sleep in your current place? When do you have to report to your new hospital? Will you be taking time off for vacation? These answers will guide your decisions for hiring a professional moving company versus enlisting friends and family. How far do you have to travel, and how many people are involved? A spouse, children, and pets will dramatically impact your entire strategy. It is relatively easy for a single person to pack a one-bedroom apartment and drive 1000 miles in a weekend. It can take a family of four weeks to move from a house in the suburbs to one just on the other side of town. Know your constraints and plan for ease and convenience. In the grand scheme of life, enjoying a leisurely move with your family is probably more important than saving a few hundred dollars on relocation costs.

Finally, prioritize what is important. Do not waste hours on minutiae when you have a limited amount of time to organize yourself before your fellowship or your first attending position. Are you trying to pack, move, and study for boards in the same four-week period? Share the burden. Delegate some responsibilities. Let the professionals take care of the moving while you prepare for the exam.

Dollars and Sense

As a resident, you learn to be thrifty. This skill will be helpful as you transition to fellowship and faculty positions. When you are planning your move, be realistic about your finances because this can be an expensive undertaking. Consider the costs of relocation in addition to the other items on your budget, such as licensure applications, board exam fees, insurance costs, and loan repayment. Meet with a financial advisor, if necessary, especially if you are purchasing a home and applying for a mortgage. Talk to your new institution about options for relocation assistance. Some Graduate Medical Education (GME) departments have funding available. New employment contracts can be negotiated to include a moving allowance, sometimes in the form of an up-front payment before you start. If you will be getting reimbursement from your employer, make sure to understand the fine print. See what they will (or will not) cover. Save receipts from the entire move. Many expenses may be tax deductible with the appropriate documentation. Keep detailed records on travel costs associated with your move. Be prepared for miscellaneous costs such as last-minute maintenance projects on your current place, professional cleaning services, utility disconnection and reconnection fees, and security deposits. Be sure to budget for years of student loans in deferment or forebearance that will go into repayment schedules as soon as you finish training.

Personal or Professional Movers?

This is an important decision for many reasons. First, the financial difference between undertaking a move yourself and hiring a company to do it for you is significant. Moving a small household a relatively short distance without professional help is certainly reasonable. Managing your own move is cheaper and gives you more control over the details; you make your own schedule. There will be no need to meet the movers in the middle of the afternoon on a Tuesday. You can decide exactly how your things are packed, which will prevent your gym shoes from winding up in the same box as your toaster. This might make unpacking slightly easier. You will worry less about how your valuables are handled when you are choosing the packing materials for your picture frames and wide-screen TV. Shop around for moving truck rentals, as this will likely be the most expensive part of moving independently. Also consider that some cities will require special permits to park large trucks or shipping containers on moving day. Please think of your moving crew if you are not using professional movers. Who is helping you move the foosball table: your buddies from Orthopedics or your parents who just applied for AARP? Can you and your friends really move a piano without professional help?

A large household, multiple family members, and a long-distance move are compelling reasons to hire a professional company. Be very thorough in searching for professional movers. Read the online customer reviews and contact references, if possible. Do not be tempted by the numerous internet offers for cheap cross-country moves by unrecognizable organizations. Large moves warrant a reputable, nationally known company. Do not compromise quality and professionalism for cost. You are entrusting all your worldly possessions to strangers for an unknown period of time and relying on them to deliver your items in a timely fashion and in the condition you left them. Lesser known companies may not function to the same standard as the giants in the industry. Dishonest companies can disregard timelines, hold your belongings hostage for higher fees, and employ questionable individuals. This headache is not worth the several hundred dollars you may have saved.

Comparison shop the larger moving companies, too. These national corporations sometimes work with local businesses. The company will send a representative to take an inventory of your things and prepare a quote. Be honest with them about the other companies you are considering because you may get a more competitive rate. Ask for any specials for students. Find out if your move will be added to a joint shipment going to the same geographic region. Be sure to discuss your rights as a client of the moving company, especially with respect to insurance and potential losses or damages to your things.

Downsizing

Moving is a perfect opportunity to declutter your life. Before investing the time and money to move certain things, take a brutally honest survey of your closet, storage spaces, furniture, and, especially, your bookshelf. Categorize all your things into three piles: keep, donate/sell, and throw away. You probably will not miss a dress you last wore in intern year. Over the course of medical school and residency, books and paper tend to accumulate and multiply. Do you need all those back issues of journals outside your specialty? Are there any USMLE or ABSITE review books you can leave in the junior resident call room?

Sometimes doing the math helps the decision to downsize. Is it more expensive to move your Ikea sofa bed across a few states or buy a new one when you get there? A quick online search can guide your options. There are countless ways to advertise and sell your furniture. Facebook, Craigslist, and community message boards are the best first step. Look into garage sales in your neighborhood or moving sales in your building. List the items you are planning to sell on a flier on campus or a private message board for residents, fellows, and students at your institution. There will always be a new class of interns and medical students looking for odds and ends for their apartments.

For anything that you cannot sell, find local organizations that accept donations. Homeless shelters and refugee centers are excellent places to drop off gently used clothes, linens, and toiletries. Habitat for Humanity may be looking for furniture in good condition. Many reputable charitable organizations will pick up kitchenware and small appliances. Consider donating to the Ronald McDonald House, women's shelters, and even your institution's ED or Trauma Center.

When it comes to the kitchen and pantry, be practical. Two weeks before a cross-country move is not the time to stock up at Costco. During the last few weeks, make creative meals with ingredients you have left rather than replenishing your fridge or freezer. Hosting a picnic or barbecue for friends and family who helped with your move is a great way to clean out the fridge and pantry. The on-call team at the hospital will happily accept leftovers. Any remaining nonperishable food items can be easily donated to the local food bank.

Before you throw something away, be conscientious. Is there someone who could use this? Many areas have recycling centers that act as a community swap for the underprivileged. Even if your town does not have these resources, a couch or a table left at the curb with a "free" sign will often find a good home.

The Survival Kit

Your survival kit is essential to a stress-free and successful move. Designate a box and/or suitcase that will travel with you instead of the movers. If you are driving your own truck, this box should be the first one you unload. Make of a list of indispensable items that you will need at your new place on the day you arrive. Include in the survival kit as much, or as little, as you like, depending on your willingness to "rough it" until your shipment arrives with the moving company or until you unpack your trailer. Be realistic and pragmatic; you can drink instant coffee until your espresso machine arrives. Stick to truly essential items for the survival kit.

Towels and toiletries should be easily accessible in the survival kit. The first thing you will be looking for when you walk into your new place is toilet paper. Another bathroom necessity is a shower curtain. Bring sleeping bags or an air mattress with a set of sheets and pillows for your first night. You will be looking forward to a good night's rest after the move. Basic kitchenware like a kettle, a small pot, flatware, and a few bowls and plates will keep you from hunting through all your kitchen boxes for those first few meals. Having a few essential necessities and may allow you to save some money on eating out until your kitchen is restocked. Candles, flashlights, and a small lamp may come in handy in spaces without built-in lighting. Tools for odd jobs (hammer, screwdrivers, pliers) will be invaluable during unpacking, connecting appliances and electronics, and inspecting existing fixtures in your new home.

Think about any personal and professional chores you will need to do during the first few weeks at your new location. Keep all the paperwork for the on-boarding process at your new institution ready at hand. Do you have the appropriate identification and credentials for official business such as opening bank accounts, closing on mortgages, and obtaining an in-state driver's license and vehicle registration? If you are taking any training courses before starting clinical work, are there any books or references that you want to have accessible? Your professional responsibilities and orientation schedule will determine the type and amount of clothes to put in your survival kit. Can you get away with shorts and flip-flops for a few days, or do you need to be prepared to have dinner with your new division chief?

Final Thoughts

Moving can be difficult, time-consuming, and expensive, but it does not have to be. Keep it all in perspective. Advance planning can eliminate most of the headaches. Recruit someone to help you organize things. That's what a mom, dad, best friend, or spouse is for! Hiring a reliable moving company will be worth the expense and convenience. Letting the professionals take care of the details allows you to focus on what is most important: savoring the experience of finally completing years of training and embarking on the next phase of your surgical career.

Chapter 19
Malpractice Pearls for the Young Surgeon

Kunal T. Vani and Matthew J. Finnegan

Introduction

Malpractice is a fact of life for physicians in the modern medical world. A *New England Journal of Medicine* article revealed that the risk of facing a malpractice claim is high. The majority of claims, however, approximately 80%, did not end up in payment to a plaintiff. A little fewer than 2% of claims end in payment to a plaintiff [1]. This article is one of the many informative ones examining the totality of the problem faced by the medical and surgical specialists. These articles do not, however, by any means, prepare you to be the defendant in a malpractice proceeding.

These facts should not overwhelm you but should challenge each and every physician to understand that these are the facts presented to us by the Institute of Medicine. These facts reveal that there are simply too many deaths related to medical mistakes, errors, or poor communication. Johns Hopkins' researchers report that medical errors rank behind heart disease and cancer as the third leading cause of death in the USA.

Based on an analysis of prior research, the Johns Hopkins study estimates that more than 250,000 Americans die each year from medical errors. Others challenge their conclusions citing the fact that existing estimates/data are not precise enough to support the above claim [2]. We believe it is clear to all who want to listen that there is a large problem with medical errors that needs to be addressed head on, in order to create a culture in medical practice that is dedicated to patient safety and preventing medical errors.

Our generation of physicians has the ability to eliminate the high number of malpractice claims by improving the quality of care we provide and buying into the

K. T. Vani, DO (✉)
General Surgery, Rowan University School of Osteopathic Medicine, Stratford, NJ, USA

M. J. Finnegan, MD, FACS
General Surgery, Lourdes Medical Associates, Haddon Heights, NJ, USA

© Springer International Publishing AG, part of Springer Nature 2018
K. Yoon-Flannery et al. (eds.), *A Surgeon's Path*,
https://doi.org/10.1007/978-3-319-78846-3_19

concept of a high reliable organization. We have personally marched for malpractice reform in Trenton, New Jersey, with thousands of physicians 20 years ago, only to see minimal reforms and high premiums stay as the norm. We as a group must improve the quality of care we provide to our patients. This alone will combat the majority of lawsuits. Safety in the hospital and physician office is paramount to the success of the physicians, nurses, and patients' outcomes.

Communication

We must ask ourselves the obvious question: how do we accomplish this daunting task? The answer is this: we must take our skills back to the bedside and connect directly with our patients, rather than relying on multiple electronic sources. One technique, lost in the computer age and often forgotten, is communication. We need to communicate better with staff, colleagues, and patients. We have come to rely heavily on nonverbal communication: text, email, Doc Halo, TigerText, etc. We have to ensure better handoff of important clinical and social information. The world of the iPhone, Internet, and electronic medical record (EMR) is here to stay, but we can soften this reality in hospital-based interaction by becoming more compassionate listeners.

Documentation

Documentation of the facts that we obtain from our patients and the discussions that we have with our colleagues are the best defensive medicine you can practice. Being vague, writing incomplete notes, and, the big favorite, reusing the same EMR note will only increase the likelihood that the court will find you at least incompetent, if not negligent. They need to prove that it is unlikely that other physicians would handle the case in the same manner. Detailed documentation can certainly help.

Always remember that the standard of care, in legal terms, is the level at which the average prudent provider in a given community setting would practice. It is how similarly qualified practitioners would have managed the patient's care under the same or similar circumstances.

If you go to radiology and discuss a CT scan with an attending radiologist, and the conclusions of the discussion will influence your management decision as whether to operate on a patient or not, you need to document this discussion in the medical record and discuss the findings with your patient. Communication, whether in person or via telephone, with other providers that are involved in changes in management should be documented. A lack of documentation in the medical record and communication to the patient or family may lead to litigation if the patient has an adverse outcome.

Malpractice Coverage

Malpractice coverage is another area where physicians need to understand not just the limits of their coverage but what type of coverage they have. Most policies have a consent clause. Make sure you read this, and whether you are an employed physician (about 60% of us) or in business for yourself or with a large group, you should be able to consent to settle or not. This means that an insurance company, or health system, cannot settle a lawsuit without your consent.

Be aware of the limits of your liability coverage. Most policies on the East Coast where we practice are one million per incident and three million per year. Some groups and health systems may pay for additional coverage for specialists in high-risk fields.

The most important item is what type of insurance you have [3]. There are currently two types of coverage: occurrence and claims-made. The difference is that occurrence policies, which are usually more expensive, will insure you no matter when the claim is made. A claims-made policy will only cover you for the period declared in the policy.

For instance, if you are covered with claims-made policy and the policy end date is June 30, and you finish your contract and move to another job, you will not be covered on July 1 for a lawsuit that occurred during the previous year unless you purchase a tail coverage. A tail coverage usually provides you coverage for all claims during the previous employment period (or dates of previous policy), but this can be very costly. It can cost up to or more than $100,000.00. If your contract doesn't specify who pays the tail, it is your responsibility. If you go uncovered, it is against the law in some states and could result in risking your personal assets. If this were the case, I would strongly recommend that you discuss asset protection with your attorney.

Don't fall into the trap of choosing to earn easy money as a young attending. By this, I mean, be wary of the many locum groups who will offer you anything to cover a weekend at the House of God Hospital in what's-your-name county, the USA. These may seem like great opportunities, but can be big malpractice traps.

In addition, remember that the data is clear that if you have been up working for 24 h straight, you may be considered legally intoxicated by some authors. Go home and rest. Your partners can handle urgent issues. Your patients will understand. Every patient deserves a well-rested surgeon.

Malpractice Rules for Physicians

Despite your best efforts, what happens if you still receive your first malpractice claim? Personally, it will feel devastating. But you must prepare yourself that this is inevitable. This will not be the worst thing to happen to you in life. Take a positive perspective, and perceive it as a learning experience.

First, don't discuss the case with everyone you know. Find a knowledgeable senior physician you trust to review the facts with you. Most of the time, you will find that what occurred is a common surgical or medical complication and may not be malpractice at all.

Second, learn what constitutes malpractice; understand the standard of care in your specialty. Take the opportunity to stay educated.

Third, obtaining the few continuing medical education (CME) credits that constitute the required amount for your recertification will never be sufficient. You must continue the reading plan that that nasty attending (that you never liked during your training) told you to start if you wanted to finish your residency. You must want to be a lifelong learner. The more up-to-date you are, the more prepared you are to prevent medical errors.

Fourth, remember you have the right in most cases to be defended by the attorney of your choice. Make sure if you are under contract with a physician group or hospital that they honor this. There are just as many average attorneys as there are average physicians. Find a reputable attorney. This can make the difference.

Fifth, once you identify the attorney of your choice, it is in your best interest to answer their calls and cooperate fully. I would suggest you do as much research as you can to assist your attorney in understanding what you did in the case and why. They will counsel you on what to do and how to testify.

Sixth, the deposition is important. Make time to prepare with your attorney. You may not remember the case by the time you get to this phase, but you must be prepared. Read the chart and discuss the details with your attorney. Discuss responses to expected questions with your attorney.

Finally, if you offer your opinion in a medical malpractice case, be mindful that you always must represent the facts of the case accurately. The ethics committees of most certification boards have produced guidelines for experts, which are well worth reading. You cannot create your own medical universe or standard of care. Don't sacrifice your principles for a few dollars. Always speak the truth and offer valid opinions.

References

1. Jena AB, et al. Malpractice risk according to physician specialty. N Engl J Med. 2011;365:7.
2. Makary MA, Daniel M. Medical error—the third leading cause of death in the US. BMJ. 2016;353:i2139. https://doi.org/10.1136/bmj.i2139.
3. Loria K. Tips for physicians to purchase the right malpractice insurance. Med Econom. 2017 Jun 10.

Chapter 20
Academic Medicine

Jonathan Nguyen and Bryan C. Morse

Introduction

Academic medicine can be one of the most rewarding fields in medicine. Academic medicine allows you to practice the art of surgery you have spent so much of your life preparing for, advance medicine, develop innovative surgical tools, and train the next generation of surgeons. Depending on your training, however, your idea of what is required to be an academic surgeon may vary.

Types of Academic Affiliations and Positions

An academic position can be at a prestigious institution, or it can start as an affiliation at a satellite hospital of a big university medical center. Depending on the agreement between you and the institution, the resources, academic responsibilities, teaching requirements, and "prestige" may vary. Types of institutions at which you hold an academic position may also vary from a university medical center to a community hospital with a recent affiliation.

A *clinical or adjunct instructor* has an association with the university and teaches students or residents, but the administrative and research obligations may not be there. This may be a community hospital that has an affiliation with the university

J. Nguyen, DO (✉)
Division of Trauma and Critical Care, Department of Surgery, Morehouse School of Medicine, Atlanta, GA, USA
e-mail: jnguyen@msm.edu

B. C. Morse, MD
Trauma/Surgical Critical Care, Department of Surgery, Grady Memorial Hospital, Emory University School of Medicine, Atlanta, GA, USA

© Springer International Publishing AG, part of Springer Nature 2018
K. Yoon-Flannery et al. (eds.), *A Surgeon's Path*,
https://doi.org/10.1007/978-3-319-78846-3_20

and takes their students and residents on rotations. Alternatively, you may be a private practice physician but happen to do cases with residents at the university hospital. In this situation, because you are engaged with the residents and students, you have gained that affiliation. While your involvement in this position is usually to provide education, there are opportunities to work with residents and students to perform clinical research based on your operative volume.

The "academic" positions we are all more familiar with are the *assistant professor, associate professor, and full professor*. These positions have associated educational, research, and administrative requirements often times in addition to a fairly busy clinical practice. Research at this level can be basic science, translational or purely clinical based on your interests—keeping in mind that if you want to do basic science research, you need to be affiliated with a laboratory as well. A key difference here (and one that should be discussed with the employer) is that your advancement is often dependent on your research productivity and your national exposure, in addition to your clinical productivity. Your ability to succeed here requires that you balance your time between the "academic" and "clinical" realms. These positions may be held at the university hospital or still at a community hospital that has heavy involvement with the parent institution. It is also important to note that salary at academic institutions may be substantially less than that of your private/community practice colleagues. In short, if you want to be affiliated with an academic center in some regard, you are not mandated to practice at a large tertiary referral center. You just have to find the right fit for you.

I Want to Be a Surgeon Scientist

So you want to be a surgeon scientist and work at the large tertiary center? That's great! There are a few things you need to know. This career requires that you balance your clinical practice with your administrative, educational, and research responsibilities. The dirty secret most people don't tell you is that your clinical practice may consume 100% of your time, but your advancement is tied to your research productivity, education, and service to the institution (defined as participation in committees and podium presentations in national organizations). In some regard, the cards are stacked against you to begin with, and the only way to succeed is to know what the requirements are ahead of time and to manage your time and resources appropriately.

1. Start with the initial interview process once you know that you and the employer are interested. Ask them what the requirements are to progress to each successive level. What tools do they have to help you reach those? How many of their current staff are hitting those marks at their years of experience? If they aren't, why not? It is important to understand that academic departments, especially surgery, tend to be hierarchal and that your first few years in practice are primarily clinical. In this sense, it is challenging to stay on track for academic promotion

because of time constraints; however, it is important to keep your goals and objectives clearly outlined and hold yourself accountable. It is very easy to get derailed and become a clinical workhorse. Having "X"% full-time equivalent (FTE) and "Y"% administrative time is great! However, how will they protect that? How will they protect that time for you to not only perform your educational and administrative duties but your research activity as well? What "administrative" duties are you required to also participate in? In the modern era, as universities are taking a hard look at the financial bottom line, administrative time may be hard to come by. Most of your FTE is covered by the clinical work that you do to pay for yourself. Administrative time is time that the department has you off the books performing some task(s) that are deemed important to them—these tasks are very limited and may be harder to justify. The best way to reduce your FTE (and make your clinical work more valuable to the department) is through research and grant support that helps pay your salary.

2. Identify your resources. Most institutions have ongoing research, and you should discuss resources before you are hired. This requires that you have an in-depth understanding of your research and education goals and anticipate things you will need to be successful. Find out what assistants they have, projects you can help complete, and projects no one has time for. One of the goals of a good chairperson or division chief is to get their faculty promoted rapidly, and they will appreciate you being proactive on this. For example, if your focus is going to be education, you may want to negotiate for the department to send you to surgeon education courses or provide you resources to teach. Similarly, if your focus is research, you may want to negotiate that the department provide you with money and time to get a master's degree in clinical research. Are there research residents and students that can help you? If the answer is no, find them. Email the residents and students to see if there is anyone interested. Also, see if there are people in other specialties or institutions who share your interest.

3. Know what you need to advance: Again, figure out what you need to move onto the next level, and make sure you hit your marks. Most starting academic physicians need several papers as the principal investigator, podium presentations, and educational works. This information is usually published on the department website.

4. As a type A person, you can't help but say yes to everything as you start your career. *Be careful of this!* Make sure you are taking on projects you can bring to completion, and, obviously, if you take on a project, *finish it.*

5. Like residency, there are lots of opportunities to get involved. Find the groups you are passionate about or the "opportunities for improvement" that others share, and work to improve your program.

6. Find a mentor. This is the last and final piece of advice. This may be a senior person in your group, your program chair, or someone you don't expect. Find that person to help you navigate the system and that has your back. It is one of the most crucial things you need whether you decide on academic or private practice.

Practicing in an academic setting is extremely rewarding. As surgeons, we have the privilege of caring for some of the sickest and most complicated patients in our community. In addition, we have the opportunity to advance medicine and shape the minds of the next generation of surgeons. In order to succeed in this environment, you need to understand the complexities of the system you are entering and manage your time to hit the benchmarks needed to progress to the next level.

Chapter 21
Hospital Employment

Thomas J. Cartolano

When graduating from a general surgery residency or a more specialized fellowship, starting the job search can be a daunting task. As healthcare continues to change, hospital employment will likely become more common. It also is important to note that depending on the surgical subspecialty or region, hospital-based employment may be the only option, whereas private practice opportunities may be extremely limited to nonexistent.

When I began my job search, the most important thing to me at the time was location. Being from the Chicago area, I wanted to return home, after being on the east coast for 7 years for training. My wife and I wanted to be closer to family. After the location was narrowed down, the types of jobs available were investigated narrowed down to what I felt would be the best fit. Hospital-based employment was the only option in my region, especially for my subspecialty and preferences in a new job.

It is important to discuss what one wants in a job. If you want to do bread and butter general surgery at a community hospital, private or hospital practice has their pros and cons. Also to note, as a new attending coming out of either a fellowship or residency, hospital-based employment may be better to gain valuable experience. Joining a private practice fresh out of training can be difficulty if referral patterns are set and the practice does not have enough business to go around.

Your subspecialty, if you have one, is also important. I am trauma and surgical critical care trained. My ideal job entailed less general and emergency general surgery and more trauma and surgical critical care. This ideal job is very difficult to find, since the majority of trauma centers in the country have limited operative trauma. Also, a private practice involving this ideal job is nonexistent. Hospital-based employment was really my only option.

T. J. Cartolano, DO
Trauma Surgery and Surgical Critical Care, Advocate Christ Medical Center, Oak Lawn, IL, USA

University of Illinois, Chicago, IL, USA

© Springer International Publishing AG, part of Springer Nature 2018
K. Yoon-Flannery et al. (eds.), *A Surgeon's Path*,
https://doi.org/10.1007/978-3-319-78846-3_21

Hospital-based employment options are many. Does one want a community hospital-based employment, a large health system group employment, or an academic position? All three of these options may be available in a specific job. In addition to these options, how are you paid and what are your requirements? Do you get a guaranteed salary with productivity bonus? Do you have to meet certain billing requirements before receiving part of your salary? Some hospital employment may involve a specific amount of calls or shifts. Did the group you are joining share patients, or is it a cutthroat hospital practice that everyone captures as many RVUs as possible? If it is an academic position, are you required to do research or publish and how much? These are the questions that should be asked when interviewing for these positions.

I am one of eight trauma surgeons in my group, under the umbrella of one of the largest physician groups in the Midwest. All eight of us are surgical critical care fellowship trained and take equal call. While some hospital-based groups may "dump" on the junior partners, we all take equal shifts and call, including my boss. This setup is rare in some practices. We are not RVU based but shift based. We are required to work a minimum amount of shifts per quarter. We do receive a bonus per quarter, but this is generated, for the most part, equally across the group of eight. We get paid extra if we get called in on our backup call nights, which is added to our quarterly bonus. We are salaried for the minimum shifts per quarter. Our main responsibilities entail surgical ICU, trauma floor, trauma, and OR coverage. These services are covered on a weekly basis with 1–2 in-house calls per week depending on what week of coverage we are on. We also cover one night a week of emergency general surgery (EGS) call, which averages one night every 1–2 months among the seven of us (our boss does not take EGS call). In addition to my weekly schedules, I am on faculty at a large university and cover the surgical ICU approximately 1 week a month.

This schedule was certainly ideal for me. It offered a small amount of general surgery and a large amount of trauma and critical care. My medical center is a very busy urban trauma center with a large amount of penetrating trauma, which allows for a large operative volume.

My hospital-based employment was a good fit for myself. My trauma group gets along great, and we have no problem having each other cover our patients. All of us have a niche in terms of our case mix, including neurosurgery and orthopedic surgery exposures, rib fixations, and the occasional omental flap for the very busy cardiovascular surgery group.

If a new grad is debating a hospital-based employment, there are some things to enquire about while interviewing:

How is your salary and bonus generated? Some jobs are based on RVU and productivity. Depending on the center, this may be fine, with a great opportunity to generate a significant amount of revenue over the salary. On the other hand, the amount of revenue you may be required to generate may not be possible, because of the amount of patients or cases you have. On top of that, you may work like a maniac, but your productivity is not compensated fairly. Personally, this is the greatest downside of a hospital-based employment. As a private practice surgeon, you may be generating a significant amount of revenue for your caseload, but as a hospital employee, you may be capped out in terms of revenue and compensation.

When interviewing for your prospective job, it is important to speak to all the members of your possible group. Are they happy? How long have each of them been employed at the facility? If you notice a high turnover rate among attendings, this can be a red flag, that either the hospital is not treating the employed physicians well or there is infighting within the group, along with poor leadership. One trauma program I won't name had a significant attending turnover, which was very concerning, mainly because of heavy-handed trauma leadership. No amount of money is worth it if your future coworkers are fighting one another, there is no trust among the group, or the leader of your department is difficult to work with. On the other hand, if the group appears happy, and/or the majority of the group has been at their job for over 3–4 years, this may be a great place to work.

Another factor to consider is who is paying your salary, along with your malpractice coverage. My salary is paid by the large physician group, along with my malpractice coverage. Some salaries are paid for by a hybrid hospital/university depending on the hospital practice you are a part of.

Look at the hospital that you want to be a part of. Does the hospital support the department you want to join, or do they make things difficult? Some hospitals do not support the department. If your partners are a good group, and get along, then the hospital support may not matter. From my personal experience, my partners are the best part of my job. If I had selfish partners, my job would be miserable. As a fairly new surgeon, I would not hesitate to call any of my seven other partners for a second set of eyes or help in the OR. My boss actually encourages it. As a trauma surgeon at my facility, we cover all vascular, thoracic, cardiac, and some urologic injuries. If we run into a problem in the OR we have never dealt with, our boss encourages us to call another member of the group before calling for a subspecialist. I've never felt intimidated to ever call for help, and as a new surgeon, this is of utmost importance. You never want to start a job where you can't get help or are chastised or put down for seeking that help.

To summarize, things to enquire about:

1. How well does the group get along, and are they happy?
2. Compensation and productivity bonuses.
3. Department and hospital support.
4. Call schedule and clinical responsibility.
5. Overall lifestyle.
6. Location and cost of living.

As a relatively new surgeon, I cannot be happier with my place of employment. My group is great, and my lifestyle is very good. I have opportunities to teach medical students and residents and also the opportunity to have an academic appointment. The most important advice I can give is to find a place where you think you will be happy. If your job is miserable, *you* will be miserable. Another pearl of wisdom is that you will learn more in your first job than you may have learned in residency. It's a whole different ball game when you go to ask your attending for help and you realize that you are the attending.

It is true that the majority of physicians will leave their first job within 3 years. The important questions to ask is why do these physicians leave their first job. When I accepted my position, my goal was not to move on in 2–3 years. Your first job doesn't have to be forever, but try to find a place where you will be happy. If you are a competitive candidate, you will have multiple options. Take the job that you feel right about, and that will offer the best environment to grow as a surgeon.

I am a firm believer in the motto "what is meant for you, won't miss you." As a surgeon, you will find a job that fits with your preferences. Don't settle for the second best. If you start your job search early, a job will be available that fits you. I have always believed in preparation and always planning ahead, and when it comes to a job, this is of utmost importance.

My advice to the new surgeon: do not settle for anything less. You are the one in demand.

Chapter 22
Lessons Learned in Private Practice

David M. Schaffzin

I once read that 75% of new physicians leave their first practice (all comers, not just surgeons). I am in that 75%. But you have to start somewhere. Every surgeon needs a first job, and at least 25% of them stay there for a long career.

The decision to be a private practitioner versus an academic surgeon may end up being a decision more about location or practicality rather than long-term goals. My wife had already been in practice in our region (Southern New Jersey) for 5 years when I was a colorectal fellow in Washington, DC. We had a child on the way, and while I had a desire to be more academic, involved in resident training, and planned to continue in clinical research, my choices regionally were very limited. Advertised jobs in colorectal included an SJ multispecialty group and a now defunct Graduate Hospital in Philadelphia that closed 2 years later. Both required general surgery call. Both already had colorectal surgeons. And neither peaked my interest. I also had a "handshake" deal with an SJ colorectal group that by my second month of fellowship, when had I called about starting contract talks, was not honored (at least I knew early on to keep looking). So, my choices were:

1. Keep looking and hope something else local opened up.
2. Accept that locally I would have to do some general surgery.
3. Interview outside our region, and my wife would have to find a job as well.
4. Find something else to do.

Fortunately an opportunity arose to take a second fellowship as a Clinical Research Fellow at Memorial Sloan Kettering Cancer Center. So by October of my fellowship year, I had a 1 year reprieve from having to choose what to do. During that year, I interviewed for academic positions in New York, Texas, Kentucky, and Georgia, and for private practice positions in southeastern Pennsylvania and the

D. M. Schaffzin, MD, FACS, FASCRS
Clinical Assistant Professor of Surgery, Drexel University College of Medicine, Philadelphia, PA, USA

St. Mary Medical Center, Center for Colon and Rectal Health, Inc., Langhorne, PA, USA

© Springer International Publishing AG, part of Springer Nature 2018
K. Yoon-Flannery et al. (eds.), *A Surgeon's Path*,
https://doi.org/10.1007/978-3-319-78846-3_22

same multispecialty group in SJ I had spoken with a year before. I also got to learn from world-renowned surgeons, operate on extremely complex patients, see some of the rarest pathology first hand you only learn about in medical school, and loved every day of my second fellowship. No regrets there.

There is one more variable you should know and that strongly affected my decision making process: my wife had already sacrificed a job in Florida with a Urology group she was recruited to join in the belief that we had a future… after *only 3 months of dating*. Talk about a leap of faith. And, to make matters worse, I already had to move to DC for a year during all of this. However, what does not break us makes us stronger. I tell my residents, particularly the two physician families, that 1 year apart, for any reason, is a challenge, but is ultimately do-able. However, having already being together for years, married for a period of time, having a child… you already have a strong bond. Separation does not break that. But to give up a job you were recruited for, to stay locally in the hopes that the person you love is committed to you for the long term… *that* is the definition of sacrifice.

So year 2 in fellowship, I now had a few offers on the table, a second child on the way, and an interesting *new* dilemma. I had the opportunity to stay a second year at MSKCC and finish a surgical oncology fellowship. So, I sat down with my (at the time pregnant) wife and we went over the pros and cons.

1. I never wanted to be more than a colorectal surgeon, so why would I want to do Surg Onc (ego, mostly).
2. If I took the fellowship I would have to move to NY for a year (I had been able to commute from NJ with rare stays in NYC over that year so far) with soon to be two kids under 2 at home and a wife who was working full time.
3. My wife *strongly suggested* that I had been a student long enough; it was time to get a job.
4. If we moved for any reason, she would be giving up an established practice to start anew, while I would be starting from scratch no matter what. Either way, we both would be starting over.
5. What was more important? Staying in Southern New Jersey/regionally or moving to be an academic?

The ultimate question became: What would I be willing to do in the short term to bide my time to attain my long-term goals? The answer, take a local job (Graduate Hospital now announced formally they were going to close) and so I joined a well-respected, long-established multispecialty group as their third colorectal surgeon. We moved to a larger house, but stayed in the region and became a two-income family. Not my initial goal, but a very conscious choice. So now, I was in a private practice, without residents, with no idea how to code or bill, or how to document appropriately, and had to make a living. Talk about a wake-up call.

You typically start out in private group practice salaried as an "Employed Physician." You may have a "production" bonus, where a percentage of your salary above your "cost" will be bonused back to you at the end of the year, or at some agreed upon interval. There are benefits and perks that the Employed physicians get that may be different from what the "Partners" get. Call may be different for the Employed Physician. Responsibilities may be different for the Employed Physician. Are you sensing a theme yet? Knowledge is power and finding out as much as humanly possible before you sign with a group is the most intelligent decision you will make. Both my residents and my wife's residents have all been royally screwed in contract negotiations, occasionally leaving them without a job, despite accepting an offer.

So what are the most valuable lessons I learned about choosing private practice?

1. Know the reputation of the group you are joining:

   (a) Find out if anyone left recently or was fired, call them as they will be "happy" to talk with you (brutally honest is another way to put it).
   (b) Take what everyone says with a grain of salt, but listen carefully.
   (c) Find out who refers to the group, and call them. Most people who like the group you will join are happy to talk them up. Conversely, those who really don't like the group will also be happy to openly speak with you.

2. Find out what "partnership" means, what path is offered to be a partner, how long will it take, and if there is a buy in.

   (a) In this day and age, buying into a practice maybe be more like throwing money away. There is the value of assets and of any real estate, but what you pay to buy in goes directly into the pockets of the partners. Know what the breakdown of any buy in might be, as much of it may be simple payment to partners for the privilege of being there, while there may be a differential in the benefits you get from being a partner for the first few years of partnership (translation, you may keep paying for the privilege of being a partner even after you are one).
   (b) Find out if the group is in negotiations to be purchased by a hospital system. More and more practices these days are being bought up, and you may join one group, but 2 years later, now work for someone else, with new rules, requirements, benefits, etc.… If you buy in to a practice, will you get bought out at the same rate as more senior partners? To paraphrase Animal Farm: All Animals Are Equal, But Some Are More Equal Than Others.

3. Hire a lawyer who specializes in contracts.

   (a) Any contract offered is to the practices benefit, NOT yours.
   (b) While many things may be nonnegotiable, make sure that every new physician is offered the same contract. If they are tailored to individuals, there may be a lot of room for negotiation. If the practice won't give your attorney other starting physicians' contracts to review, this may be a sign they cannot be trusted.
   (c) Remember, attorneys work on hourly rates (include fees per phone call, per email, and bill in 0.25 h, etc.…). Fees can become astronomical.
   (d) Remember, attorneys work for *you*. They often have secondary gain issues, like billable hours. Do not let them go overboard on things they *think* you deserve, when no one else at that practice has that benefit. It may be $20,000 or more later before you find out that some things in the contract cannot be changed.

4. Make sure the practice you are joining has a contact person (a physician) you can speak with directly. Many issues can be resolved easily by talking directly with your new group instead of through lawyers. You are a physician, a professional, and hopefully planning a long-term career with the group. The process should be open and transparent. If the group is hiding things from you, they probably will continue to do so once you are employed. But an honest negotiation includes telling them your fears, and not letting them take advantage of you.

I hope you found this helpful. I did ultimately leave that group... but that is another story.

Part III
After Finding a Job

Chapter 23
Partners

Marc Neff

Introduction

When you enter into a surgical residency, you quickly realize that you spend more time in the hospital than out of it. That leads to some interesting changes and challenges in your relationships. Spending 12 or more hours a day with people day in and day out, and they start to become your friends and family, your confidants, and sometimes even lead to intimate relationships. This chapter isn't meant to pass any judgment on who you spend your time with in the hospital, or out of the hospital; it is merely meant to raise the awareness that these relationships with your partners, whether work or personal, are complicated by your life as a surgeon.

Business Partners

Partners at work are the closest to understanding what you are really dealing with day in and day out. They will see your office schedule. They will know how complex the patients are you see on rounds. They will understand the challenges of dealing with the difficult family. They will be named in the same malpractice cases. They have the same pressures for productivity. They have the same call schedule issues. They have the same issues with the inane resident calls in the middle of the night. They understand how much you struggled to dig that tumor out of the pelvis, and they know how exhausting it is to teach the second year resident on probation. They know the pressures of getting home on time for dinner and recognize the pain of the electronic health records (EHR) and endless paperwork. Because they understand all this, it's important to appreciate them, to say thank you, to be honest with

M. Neff, MD, FACS, FASMBS
Center for Surgical Weight Loss, Jefferson Health New Jersey, Cherry Hill, NJ, USA

© Springer International Publishing AG, part of Springer Nature 2018
K. Yoon-Flannery et al. (eds.), *A Surgeon's Path*,
https://doi.org/10.1007/978-3-319-78846-3_23

them, and to be open and communicative. Don't make their job any more difficult than it already is. Just like your brother or sister, if you support them, they will support you. Of course you can disagree with them, challenge them, and even get mad and yell at them. But then, you have to essentially kiss and make up. You and your partners are a team, day in and day out. If you aren't a unified front, the whole group collapses from the onslaught of the outside world that is the hospital. Communicate with your partners often. You may sometimes feel alone, but you can always call your partner to bail you out, help you out, discuss a complex case with, or get their input or advice. If you aren't able to do this, you have to consider if you have the right business partners.

Personal Partners

I've added personal partners to this chapter to emphasize something very important. You will spend more awake time with your work colleagues than your life partner. That means you have to put more effort into your relationship outside of the hospital. Your spouse and family won't understand the pressures of your job and won't understand why you need to see your postoperative patient with the anastomotic leak first thing in the morning, every morning. They won't understand why you are late for dinner or in answering pages or texting during family outings. They won't understand why you spend so much time giving your attention to perfect strangers when they are supposed to be your priority. The message here is plain; the time you have outside of the hospital with your spouse and family has to be high-quality time. You can't come home exhausted and not participate. You can't blame your bad mood on what happened at work. Leave it there. Be present. You work hard to provide for your family, but an equally important part is to be able to share in the enjoyment with them of what that work provides for. You aren't simply a workhorse. Believe me, your family wants you present. And after enough time of not being present, your family will go on without you.

Chapter 24
Medical Economics

Alan M. Neff

The W's: Who, What, and Why

Healthcare economists are not that different than any other economists, and in general we all like to think about the same things. These include the effects of new technology, how services and products get priced, antitrust policy that keeps prices down and competition fair, what the appropriate level of private and public investment should be, and strategic behavior—the actions taken that affect the overall market. In healthcare we think about these things in terms of the following actors—individual consumers or patients, providers, manufactures including medical device manufacturers and pharmaceutical companies, public and private organizations, and finally federal, state, and local governments.

Here's the part where everyone's eyes glaze over. We study these things in terms of those actors using tools like theories of production, efficiency, disparities, competition, scarcity, marginal analysis, distinctions between "needs" and "wants," opportunity cost, equity, and, everyone's favorite, supply and demand.

We study these things so we can tell governments which laws and regulations to pass. We also advise device manufacturers and pharmaceutical companies on which new health inventions, systems, or services will produce the best and, yes, most profitable outcomes. We also try to predict consumer and provider responses to changes in public policy and incentives provided by governments.

See? It is not so different from all other economics, *except* for the extensive government intervention, the uncertainty because we're talking about something that's hard to measure called "health," the information gap between patients and providers, the barriers to entry, the presence of third-party agents (insurers), and the screwy purchasing model where the physician makes purchases for the patient (consumer) without knowing the cost [1].

A. M. Neff, MBA, HCM
Neuro Diagnostic Devices, Prescott, AZ, USA

© Springer International Publishing AG, part of Springer Nature 2018
K. Yoon-Flannery et al. (eds.), *A Surgeon's Path*,
https://doi.org/10.1007/978-3-319-78846-3_24

It's Just Supply and Demand, Stupid

In 1972 Michael Grossman did the first serious work on how economists should think about consumer behavior regarding healthcare. "The central proposition of the model is that health can be viewed as a durable capital stock that produces an output of healthy time. A person determines his optimal stock of health capital at any age by "equating the marginal efficiency of this capital to its user cost in terms of the price of gross investment" [2]. That sounds like a great way to think about how patients decide to spend their healthcare dollars if only consumers actually spent their healthcare dollars. One problem is that consumers don't buy healthcare; they buy insurance. For simplicity, let's include the deductible in the cost of the insurance. Other than a small co-payment, a patient's cost for healthcare services is essentially zero. Thus, the return on the patient's "investment" is almost infinite regardless of how small the marginal benefit in his or her health. This is really, really bad. Imagine a world of drivers where there were $24 co-pay per accident after you paid your deductible each year. And you got paid for your time off from work for each accident or if you had a really bad accident you could apply for government assistance. No one would have an incentive to be "careful" when they drove. I, for one, would be afraid to drive. The patient or consumer generates a very flat (or as we economists call it "inelastic") demand curve where the consumer essentially has an insatiable appetite for more healthcare services (their demand is very insensitive to changes in price since there price is essentially zero). With a "normal" good or service, the demand curve slopes downward, meaning that as the price increases, the consumer demands less.

In this world where there is essentially no limit on patient demand, you can see why the market generated a "fee-for-service" (FFS) model. If the market continued to pay to keep a patient "healthy" (capitation), it would quickly run out of services.

Let's digress for a moment to see how we got into this mess. Before 1942 less than 9% of the population had health insurance. Baylor hospital in Texas started looking for ways to get people to pay for hospital stays. For 50 cents per month, they offered to cover a person's hospital stay. During the great depression, no one could afford to privately pay for a hospital stay so the Baylor model took off—eventually becoming known as Blue Cross. In order to assuage the inflation accompanying WWII, Congress passed the "Stabilization Act of 1942," which included wage and price controls [3]. As a concession to workers whose wages were frozen, the Act allowed businesses to offer insurance plans, including health insurance plans, as a fringe benefit. In 1943 the IRS ruled that employer-based health insurance should be tax-free [4]. Soon Blue Cross was everywhere, and by the 1960s about 70% of the population was covered by some form of health insurance.

We have "evolved" from the days when just hospitalization or catastrophic healthcare was covered by insurance and consumers covered their own day-to-day healthcare costs to the model today where *everything* is covered. And as we've discussed, when lunch is free, then people start to order lunch throughout the day.

If the consumer actually had to pay for each healthcare service they received, the demand curve would be downward sloping—they would demand fewer healthcare services as the price increased, and they would also demand less expensive alternatives. One of these alternatives is to lead a healthier lifestyle. Grossman would say that they are reallocating their healthcare dollars to maximize the return on their healthcare stock.

Demand Is Not the Only Stranger in Town

Given how perverse the demand curve is, you would think that healthcare is complicated enough. Sorry, no such luck. Since hospitals cannot increase their supply of beds without substantial capital investment and surgeons cannot simply perform more surgeries if you double their salaries and pharmaceutical companies pay an average of $2.6 billion to research and develop each new drug which takes about 10 years, the supply curve for healthcare is very steep (inelastic) [5]. That means for any given change in price, the supply of healthcare services does not change very much. And that is what makes healthcare economics so difficult a subject to think about. Consumers have an insatiable appetite for services, and the system has a fixed supply of services (at least in the short run). So how does the Affordable Care Act stuffing 24 million more people into the system improve things? [6] That's an excellent question.

ACA Goals and Reality

The theory behind the Affordable Care Act was to push off government-provided services, which they were never good at providing, into the private market, which has a history of providing more effective services at a lower cost. In theory everyone is better off. But the cost savings have not flowed down to the consumer. And while the insurers have gotten richer, healthcare has gotten more expensive and consumers have even fewer choices.

Many argue that we are approaching a tipping point where people just opt out of the insurance system altogether and choose to pay privately for their healthcare. Isn't that where we started in the 1920s? Welcome to the revolution! One distinct possibility is that all of this implodes into a single-payer system or some form of socialized medicine. That's bad for the people without money who will suffer from decreased access and regulated supply. The rich, well, they always find a way—in this case it's called concierge medicine, and it's already here. Plastic surgery has already undergone such a transformation. While some procedures are covered by insurance, plastic surgeons have generally switched to a cash-pay business model.

"In the Long Run, Everything Is a Toaster"

Bruce Greenwald taught a value-investing course at Columbia Business School. "In the long run," he says, "everything is a toaster." In other words, all great innovations eventually become commodities, bought on the basis of price and nothing else [7]. We already see this in the FFS model. Since hospitals cannot change the number of beds in the short run, since surgeons cannot clone themselves to perform more surgeries, and since pharmaceutical companies cannot bypass the FDA to produce more drugs quicker, the natural response is to break down existing services into even smaller units. If the providers (suppliers) can make the sum of the revenue from those individual units greater than what they were charging for the entire service in the past, then they increase their profits.

The government fight against this trend started with a new payment model proposed by the ACA called an Accountable Care Organization (ACO). According to Centers for Medicare and Medicaid Services (CMS), an ACO is a group of doctors, hospitals, and other healthcare providers who join voluntarily to give coordinated high-quality care to their Medicare patients. Of the original 32 ACOs created, less than 20 survive today. But CMS is pushing back and announced that by 2018 their goal is to have 50% of Medicare patients enrolled in an ACO (or some other form of bundled payment system) and that 90% of their claims would be processed that way. CMS is doing its best to move away from the FFS model. But in an industry where most of the providers know nothing else except FFS, can that ever happen?

Conclusion

What does this all mean? Because patients do not have the same knowledge as healthcare providers, healthcare is largely a "want" rather than a "need," and because of previous government intervention in line with making healthcare a "right," we have generated an infinite "want." By restricting pharmaceutical companies, hospitals, physicians, and other healthcare providers in the name of "safety" or "fairness," we have artificially restricted the supply. We have screwed up the supply and demand curves so much that the market cannot resolve itself. What is the hope for an infinite "want" being satisfied by an artificially restricted supply?

The only solution will come from changing the demand and supply curves. We change the supply curve through innovation in medicine that increases the supply of healthcare. Adding 24 million people to the insurance roles doesn't accomplish anything unless you change the shape of the supply curve or move it to the right. Innovations like shorter development times for new drugs, longer patent protections, or tax breaks for developing orphan drugs help move the supply curve to the right. More models where primary care is provided by nurse practitioners and physician assistants are supervised by physicians also move the supply curve. More alternatives to nursing homes include adult day care, home care, accessory dwelling units (ADUs), subsidized senior housing, board and care homes, continuing care retirement communities (CCRCs), respite care, and Programs of All-Inclusive Care for the Elderly (PACE) are needed. And while we change the supply curve, we must also change the demand curve by challenging the concept that healthcare is a pure "right" with no real cost associated with it and that patients (consumers) have no responsibility for maintaining their own "health." We must change the demand and supply curves; everything else just makes us feel better about ourselves. And that's not healthcare.

References

1. Phelps CE. Health economics. 3rd ed. Boston: Addison Wesley; 2003.
2. Grossman M. On the concept of health capital and the demand for health. J Polit Econ. 1972;80(2):223–55.
3. Stabilization Act of 1942. Pub.L. 77–729, 56 Stat. 765, enacted October 2, 1942.
4. https://economix.blogs.nytimes.com/2013/07/30/the-question-of-taxing-employer-provided-health-insurance/?_r=0
5. http://phrma-docs.phrma.org/sites/default/files/pdf/rd_brochure_022307.pdf
6. http://obamacarefacts.com/sign-ups/obamacare-enrollment-numbers/
7. Michael Schrage. The myth of commoditization. Magazine: Winter 2007 Opinion & Analysis 2007 Jan 01. http://sloanreview.mit.edu/article/the-myth-of-commoditization/

Chapter 25
Gifts

Marc Neff

As a surgeon, it is easy to get lost in the number of procedures we do. The average general surgeon, in some locals, will do 500+ surgeries a year. That makes it hard to distinguish one gallbladder from another. However, it sure is nice to be appreciated. I have a collection of cards and gifts that patients have given me. I even have a monogrammed briefcase that a pharmaceutical rep gave me in residency. While most gifts are truly given from the heart, there is much more scrutiny in today's world, and the concern for bribes and coercion is real.

The American Medical Association (AMA) website has statements regarding accepting or declining gifts. It is worth a review. While most are an expression of gratitude, there is a real concern that must always be present, which is the patient trying to influence care or secure preferential treatment. The code of medical ethics concerning gifts requires that physicians should:

- Be sensitive to the gifts' value and the timing of the gift
- Not allow the gift to influence medical decision-making or patient care

An easy litmus test here is would you feel embarrassed to share news of the gift with your partners, colleagues, staff, or family. If so, then declining the gift in a sensitive way can be offered. An out may be to suggest a charitable contribution instead. While some physicians take the position of never accepting gifts, the rejection of a gift that leaves the givers feeling hurt, rejected, or financially impacted can damage the doctor-patient relationship. Be aware of your organizations and hospital/group policies. Many have a limit above which gifts have to be reported (often around $50).

Gifts from pharmaceutical and instrument companies have long been an issue for physicians. This was the topic of a paper published in 1991 by the AMA, *Gifts to Physicians From Industry* [1]. Similar papers have been published by the American

M. Neff, MD, FACS, FASMBS
Center for Surgical Weight Loss, Jefferson Health New Jersey, Cherry Hill, NJ, USA

© Springer International Publishing AG, part of Springer Nature 2018
K. Yoon-Flannery et al. (eds.), *A Surgeon's Path*,
https://doi.org/10.1007/978-3-319-78846-3_25

College of Physicians [2]. The conclusions of these published guidelines were that gifts are permitted if they are:

- Not of substantial value
- Benefit the patient
- Related to the physicians' practice
- For office use, patient care, or education

So, in conclusion, use your best judgment. An intimate gift or extravagant gift is clearly out of bounds. But most gifts fall into a gray area. Ask yourself why the gift was given. Does it make you feel good? Does it influence the care you deliver? Can you share the disclosure of the gift comfortably with your family and other health-care professionals?

References

1. Council on Ethical and Judicial Affairs of the American Medical Association. Gifts to physicians from industry. JAMA. 1991;265:501.
2. American College of Physicians. Physicians and the pharmaceutical industry. Ann Intern Med. 1990;112:624–6.

Chapter 26
Marketing

Steven M. Pandelidis

Growing up as the son of a Greek immigrant psychiatrist and an American-born pharmacist of Greek heritage, I was well aware of what it means to be part of a medical family. From my parents, I learned about the need for long hours and dedication on the part of my father but also the importance of a charming mother who helped my father navigate the social strata of the local medical community. My parents had their Greek friends and their doctor friends. Being fully engaged with the other doctors on a social level as well as involvement with hospital committees, the local medical society and hospital governance were the key to my father's success. Of course long hours at work and tremendous commitment to his patients were essential.

The training in surgery in this country is of the highest quality, so to distinguish oneself from the competition, a surgeon has to make a special effort. For the most part, an individual surgeon is not easily distinguished from their colleagues. The secret is convincing your referring physicians that you are unique. The quality of the work one does will certainly slowly distinguish a surgeon. Early on, the surgeon should focus on maximizing patient and referring physician interactions. For example, I volunteered for extra call in my private group, and I always made room for one more new patient in my practice.

It is most helpful to have a niche, which separates you from others. I am a general surgeon/surgical oncologist. My training in surgical oncology was excellent, but we certainly had an emphasis in melanoma and head and neck surgery. I recognized when I started my first job that nobody routinely took care of melanoma patients, so there was an opportunity to distinguish myself. The ENT physicians had a bit of a lock on the treatment of smoking-induced head and neck cancers, and a soon-to-be retiring plastic surgeon did the majority of thyroid/parathyroid surgeries. Recognizing the opportunity in the landscape, I immediately set out to establish myself as the primary melanoma and endocrine surgeon.

S. M. Pandelidis, MD
WellSpan Surgical Oncology, York, PA, USA

Soon after starting my first job, I made a point of calling every dermatologist as well as every endocrinologist in my medical community. I not only visited them in their offices, but I also took them all out to dinner. Over the years, I never stopped this practice. When a new potential physician came to town, I would contact them. I became friends with my medical colleagues. They also understood that their offices had a direct "bat phone" to my practice. More recently, in the last decade, all of these physicians have my cell numbers. My secretary simply understands that if we get a call from the dermatologists or the endocrinologist, that patient is seen within the next few days. If the doctor needs to call me, they can call me in the OR or the office, and I will drop what I'm doing (if possible) and speak to them. It is not unusual that my circulating nurse holds the phone up to my ear in the OR so I can speak to my colleagues. Often, the OR staff will stare at me in disbelief, and I turn to them and say, "That's how you build a practice."

Whenever you get a call from a colleague, always get their cell phone number and put it in your phone, and volunteer your number to any colleague. Availability is paramount!

Once you are fortunate enough to get a referral, make sure your correspondence with the physician is prompt and worthwhile. Do not send a perfunctory EMR note, which looks more like an itemized bill or population health document than a legitimate colleague-to-colleague communication. Early on in practice, my correspondence was a separate dictated letter with "just the facts, ma'am." I'm certain the family doctor is not interested in my heart and lung exam or their patient's medication list.

Now, with EMR all of my correspondence to the referring physician begins with a typed message by me complete with misspellings and punctuation errors, so it is obvious I typed it myself. If you type it yourself, you choose your words more carefully. The rest of the note may be my EMR gibberish to justify evaluation/management (E&M) codes and to satisfy all regulations.

As an example:

Dear Dr. Tons of patients or Dear Jack (if I know them well enough),
We will plan wide excision and sentinel node biopsy for Mrs. Jones' 2.4 mm L arm
melanoma. There is an 18% chance of a + node. If the node is negative, the cure
rate is 92%. Once we get her through her operation, I will thereafter follow her
per NCCN guidelines for life.
Thx
Steve P

The referring physician can then read three lines and know that their patient is in good hands. If they are not yet convinced, they will also receive a similarly simple but informative follow-up letter updating them with the outcome of the operation as well as intraoperative pictures if appropriate (Fig. 26.1). There are plenty of capable surgeons, but if one sends a quality picture of a quality operation, you may have a loyal referring physician for the length of your professional career.

Fig. 26.1 Intraoperative, quality picture of a parotidectomy

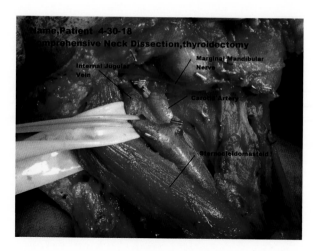

If your patient is a cancer patient, every time you see that patient, you will send an update to the referring physician which hopefully begins with a positive message that the patient is seen and there is no evidence of recurrence. In 5 sentences the referring physician knows his/her patient is fine and moves on to the next note in his or her dreaded task folder.

Never take your referring physicians for granted. Meet the new ones but always let your established colleagues know how much you appreciate their trust.

Chapter 27
Finding a Mentor

Marc Neff

It may seem a little strange to have a chapter that focuses on finding a mentor after residency is over, but the truth is, this is so incredibly valuable. At every stage in our training, we need guidance. As a medical student learning how to close our first wound, to the young research attending applying for a research grant or encountering their first malpractice case, having a mentor to guide you through the hurdles you will face will make those hurdles easier.

This is a hard lesson to learn, the value of mentorship. Many residents think too highly of themselves to feel like they need help. Some may feel too insecure to feel comfortable admitting that they need help. The idea of asking for help as an attending is even harder. The truth is that we all need help, at every stage in our lives. No one has it all figured out. The wisdom and life experiences of those who went before you can save you from making the same mistakes. I believe it is mentioned elsewhere in this book, but the lesson is repeated every week at our mortality and morbidity conference. "Wisdom comes from experience, the best wisdom, from the worst experience. And it is better to learn it from someone who has already had the experience than to experience it yourself."

I'm not suggesting that everyone out there is going to find the perfect mentor to help them through every struggle as a surgical attending from personal life to work challenges to learning new techniques and publishing research. What I am suggesting, however, is that it is worth it to take the time to assemble a group of mentors and think of them as such to cover most aspects in your life. You will find older attending to be very receptive to giving back. You will be able to find the senior department chair that can mentor you on how the politics of the hospital works and the tenured professor that can teach you on grants. You'll find the recently divorced surgeon who can teach you about relationships and the attending with five children that can teach you how to balance home life, school schedules, and making lunches.

M. Neff, MD, FACS, FASMBS
Center for Surgical Weight Loss, Jefferson Health New Jersey, Cherry Hill, NJ, USA

© Springer International Publishing AG, part of Springer Nature 2018
K. Yoon-Flannery et al. (eds.), *A Surgeon's Path*,
https://doi.org/10.1007/978-3-319-78846-3_27

People like to talk about themselves and their experiences, and all it takes is a drop of curiosity and you can save yourself hours of struggling to make a call schedule, when someone already knows all the tricks; save yourself many sleepless nights about your upcoming deposition for your malpractice case when you can speak to someone who has been through it several times. Not all the information you will get will be valuable, and some of the information will undoubtedly be specific to their situation, but I can think of very few times I have sat with a senior attending and asked them an open question about their area of expertise and not come away with a kernel of wisdom that would have been a painful or time-consuming lesson to learn. Do you really want to spend the time figuring out the best ways to attract referrals? Spend way too much money on marketing that a more senior surgeon knows will never work? Just like asking for directions when you start at a new hospital, finding a mentor you can ask for advice when you face a new challenge can help you from getting lost.

Chapter 28
Setting Up Your Office

John D. Paletta

Introduction

Upon completion of residency and fellowship, most physicians will enter some form of clinical practice, which will inevitably require an office. Specific involvement and input in the establishment of this office varies depending on the type of practice proposed. Entering a solo private practice will afford complete autonomy and sole responsibility, which can be rewarding but also time-consuming. Other practice situations including small group, large group, multi-specialty, academic, or hospital employee groups will involve less time and input but also less control overall. No matter what type of practice you will ultimately decide on, you can and should have input on many aspects of setting up your office.

Achieving a successful practice, or even defining a "successful practice," does not follow a specific blueprint. To a certain degree, your financial situation will force some decisions regarding necessities versus luxuries in your work environment. A harmonious working environment will evolve with time and experience. This broad overview introduces many of the issues involved in setting up an office, which may not apply in every situation. Mistakes on both medical and business decisions are inevitable, and it is not the end of the world. Learn from them and continue to grow.

Physical Office Space

With so many aspects to setting up a successful office, consider some questions regarding the physical space that you would like your office to occupy.

J. D. Paletta, MD, FACS
The Georgia Institute for Plastic Surgery, Savannah, GA, USA

© Springer International Publishing AG, part of Springer Nature 2018
K. Yoon-Flannery et al. (eds.), *A Surgeon's Path*,
https://doi.org/10.1007/978-3-319-78846-3_28

Where will your office be located in proximity to the hospitals that you will cover?

Location, location, location. This is an important consideration from a time management standpoint. Your office should be strategically located to allow you to quickly check on patients or see consults with minimal disruption to your office practice. Always try to minimize travel time in order to maximize efficiency. Most hospitals have a professional building on campus or nearby that would be a great option for your office space. Privately owned office complexes that are largely medical are often close to hospitals as well. A readily accessible location is important so patients can easily find you, and certain specialties benefit from walk-in business (e.g., cosmetic procedures such as Botox, fillers, hair removal, vein treatments, etc.).

Will you rent or own the physical office space?

Initially starting a solo practice, you will most likely rent a physical space in order to preserve cash and minimize debt. Incurring a large mortgage at the start may hamper your ability to become profitable in a timely manner and grow your business. If you choose to rent, make certain that the terms of the contract are not so limiting that you are locked in to a specific location for a long period of time. You may find that your initial location is not ideal, and flexibility will afford you the ability to adapt your practice in a positive manner.

If you join an existing practice, you will be charged rent by the owners of the physical space, who may even be your new business partner(s). Always make certain that the rent for the physical space is reasonable and appropriate for the area and that you understand the provisions in your contract regarding the upkeep of the physical space. If the building needs paint, or a new roof, or even updated landscaping, who will be responsible for the repairs?

Finally, make sure that your office space has room to expand with your growing business. It may be better to pay for a larger space than is initially required than to move your practice in a year when you outgrow your physical space.

What will your sign look like, and where will it be located?

Consider signage as well as location. Your office should be attractive from the outside as well as the inside, and the sign for the practice is the first impression for your patients. Make sure it is not only attractive and professional but also easily located from the street.

Does your proposed physical space have adequate parking for both patients and staff?

Fighting for a parking space makes for a frustrated patient before they even walk through your front door. Make sure that your parking situation is adequate for your initial patient load and allows for growth so that you do not find yourself in the position of outgrowing your space in 6–12 months as your practice (hopefully) grows.

Is your proposed physical space in compliance with local ordinances and ADA requirements?

Check on local zoning and ordinance requirements for your proposed physical location. Additionally, there are provisions in the Americans with Disabilities Act of 1990 that you must consider before you commit to a physical space. Non-compliance with these regulations may result in costly remedies or even cause you to have to abandon a physical space and start search for a physical space all over again.

Furniture and Fixtures

There are many aspects to consider when it relates to furnishing your office space, because there are many different areas that make up a physician's office. Consider your personal office, patient waiting room, employee office space, employee break areas, exam rooms, and operating room facilities. Each area is distinct and requires a specialized type of furnishing.

Your Private Office Space

Whether you join an existing group or set out on your own, you will have to furnish and decorate your private office space. Consider what tasks you complete in this space when deciding how to furnish the area. Will this be a place where you complete charts, review records, and make phone calls, or will you be seeing patients in your private office space as well?

Many physicians see patients in their private office before moving them into a room to perform a physical exam. If this will be the case in your practice, the private office area may need to be furnished with a more polished look than if it were solely a more utilitarian space.

Patient Waiting Room

First impressions are important in your new practice, and the patient waiting room is their first glimpse of your practice, a reflection on you personally as well. Furnishing the waiting area is tricky in that it should be tasteful and tidy and also able to hold up to the wear and tear that comes with the territory.

Commercial furniture is expensive and somewhat underwhelming in appearance but will hold up to the abuse that your patients will inevitably inflict. Darker fabrics are usually good choices, and spending the extra amount for stain-resistant fabrics will pay off over time. Everyone loves a luxurious waiting room, but consider your fine antique pieces being subjected to a few toddlers, and suddenly a more utilitarian room makes sense. You can make it tasteful without worrying that it will be ruined in 2 months.

Employee Office Space

Consider the office staff working space carefully when furnishing your office. Not only should these furnishings be specific to their use, but also they should be sturdy and capable of expansion if the need arises. Consider not only esthetics but comfort as well in these areas—your employees will thank you for it.

If your practice is not converted to EMR, you will need adequate storage areas, with room to grow. Off-site storage of records can be costly and cumbersome when you need to get a specific record in your hands. A well-organized office space is paramount when many employees will access stored charts and other items.

Employee Break Areas

If you do not want your employees to eat their lunch at their desks, you will most likely provide them with an area to congregate and take their lunch break. An easily cleaned area with specific zones will make your life easier in the long run.

A table and chairs, small kitchen area with sink, refrigerator, and microwave may be all you need to provide, and a policy of cleaning up after yourself is always a great plan! Having a specific space for these activities will save your employee office space from becoming a cafeteria and keep the professionalism of your office intact.

Exam Rooms

Exam rooms will need to be furnished with an exam table, a chair, and a stool. A writing space or counter of some type may be useful depending on the nature of your practice. Consider the need for medical supplies when furnishing your exam rooms, and plan the physical space accordingly. This equipment can be quite expensive, but there are ways to cut costs when setting up your office. There are vendors that sell used and refurbished exam room equipment that will make this process less painful and get you on your way to achieving a successful practice. With expanding use of technology in exam rooms, consider how this will fit into your room. You may not have much of a choice, but think about where a computer might be located compared to the exam table or the patient. With computers and technology come the necessary outlets to utilize these things, so think about this, especially if you are setting a brand new office space.

Operating Room Facilities

If your office will incorporate an operating room, this specialized equipment can be very costly as well. In addition to all of the medical equipment, specialized lighting and backup generator equipment are also a necessary part of the operating room.

Get to know the maintenance people at the hospital who repair the OR tables. You will inevitably encounter issues with your equipment, and they will serve as a valuable resource to repair your equipment as well.

Computer and Phone Equipment

Computer and phone system equipment can be very costly and highly specialized. It is a good idea to hire a consultant or person of expertise in this specific area because mistakes in acquiring the proper equipment can be very expensive to correct. The amount of hardware and software available specifically for the medical field is vast, and because it is constantly evolving, any attempt at recommendations would be obsolete before this book is even published.

Take advantage of the multitude of experts/salesmen in this area—trust me, there will be no shortage of them! There are, however, a few questions to consider before meeting with an IT professional or salesman.

Will you be utilizing EMR and tying-in to a hospital system?

Electronic medical records are the systematized collection and storage of patient information in a digital format that can be shared across different health-care settings and even accessed by patients via patient portal. If you are starting a practice from the ground up, this method of record keeping will make your life easier. If, however, you are joining an existing practice that is not currently utilizing EMR or thinking of using paper charts for patient information storage, converting to this system after the fact can be costly and time-consuming. If you choose not to utilize an EMR system, keep in mind that you will need a transcriptionist to convert dictation to hard copy format for your files.

Will you maintain your own internal IT and telephone system or hire someone to maintain it for you?

Information technology systems and specialized telephone systems change and evolve over the life of your business, and keeping up with the current systems can be a full-time job in itself. Consider whether you have the time or expertise to maintain these systems or whether you will need a professional to handle them for you.

Software and hardware must be maintained and updated, and the security of protected health information and ransomware can be very expensive if your system becomes the victim of a compromise. Assigning someone else the responsibility of maintaining the integrity of your computer system may be well worth the cost in the long run.

Will you develop and maintain a website for your practice?

A website can be a very effective tool for your practice if designed properly and an Achilles heel if designed poorly. Web designers can help you put together a great-looking website for a reasonable fee that will go a long way in patient outreach and information dissemination. You can even provide access to patient portals and patient forms for download on your website, which can save time and effort for your office staff.

Decide if you will design and maintain your own website or will enlist the help of a web designer. If you are not an expert in this area, investing the money in a professional will be a huge time-saver and will help to present your practice in a very professional and polished way.

Medical Supplies

Outfitting your office with the medical supplies necessary for patient care can be costly and a bit overwhelming. A good supply manager can make sure that you have adequate supplies on hand to meet the everyday demands of your practice, but establishing what those demand may be will take a bit of trial and error—hopefully not too much error! Here are some tips to make the process a bit less intimidating:

Develop a list of supplies that you may need available in each exam room and those that are less critical and can be kept in a central location for use as necessary.

It is not necessary to have every exam room completely stocked. In order to save on inventory expense, it is completely acceptable to have some items in a container that will travel to different exam rooms and just stock the basics in each individual room.

For instance, gauze, tape, bandages, syringes, needles, basic instruments (scissors, pick-ups, scalpels, and staple removers), and medications (alcohol, betadine, local anesthetic) will need to be readily available. The more commonly used items can be stocked in the exam rooms, while the less used items can be stored in a central location and can be quickly retrieved as needed.

Will you need patient gowns and exam table covering for examinations?

You will likely need patient gowns for examinations and clean covering for your exam tables. Keep in mind that although your patients might appreciate the cloth/linen gowns and coverings, they are very expensive and add the addition of a linen service to your growing list of expenses. Paper gowns and covering materials are less expensive and disposable. The cloth variety is definitely a nice touch but can be added down the road as your practice grows and becomes more profitable.

Will you shop for the best medical supply prices or utilize an advisory service to do the legwork for you?

There are comprehensive medical/surgical supply procurement advisory services available that will shop for the best deals on equipment and supplies that your practice needs. They make money by saving you money and are paid as a percentage of your savings. It is a win-win to employ such a service with the high cost and high volume of supplies that your practice will use and saves you the time of tracking down a good deal that might change overnight.

These types of services might not be available initially when setting up your practice, but as you establish a purchasing history, they will want your business. This is a great way to keep your overhead from getting out of control without using any of your time.

Personnel

Making good personnel decisions can be tricky, and bad decisions can be both costly and frustrating. Taking the time to evaluate personnel carefully will pay off in the end with a staff that is cohesive, qualified, and dependable. There is nothing worse than finding that you have inadequate or incompetent staff when you are trying to get your practice off the ground.

Staff can be broken down into three categories: clinical staff, business staff, and maintenance staff. Clinical staff includes personnel such as the PA, NP, RN, LPN, scrub tech, and medical assistant. Business staff includes personnel such as an office manager, billing clerks, accounts payable, accounts receivable, front desk/reception staff, phone operator, personal secretary/scheduler, insurance coordinator, and medical records clerk. Maintenance staff includes a reputable medical cleaning crew that will clean your offices after hours and properly dispose of medical waste.

A few points to consider when considering personnel for your medical practice:

Although personnel is a must item, the amount of personnel that you employ is flexible.

As personnel is very likely going to constitute the largest portion of your expenses, try to be "lean and mean" early on if your staff can handle multitasking. The name of the game is to minimize expense without sacrificing quality or patient care. You can add more staff as your practice grows and the need presents itself.

When you are just starting out, you will not need as much clinical staff as you might think.

Justifying the expense of a physician extender such as a physician assistant or nurse practitioner will be difficult until your practice becomes profitable enough to support the large salary that such personnel will demand. Remember, the larger the draw on your practice financially, the longer it will take to pull you out of debt.

You will need a nurse to perform certain duties such as patient calls, drawing up medication, and calling in prescriptions. You may not, however, require a full-time nurse. Sharing a nurse with a partner or finding a nurse who only wants to work part-time may be options to keep your overhead in check. A medical assistant will only cost half as much as a nurse and can help you when you are seeing patients and fill in when your nurse is not working. You do not have to sacrifice quality when handling these decisions as long as you are organized and schedule your staff appropriately.

Your business staff can multitask until the volume of your practice warrants dedicated personnel.

The business office is a place where multitasking makes sense early on. You will most likely be able to utilize staff in this area to wear more than one hat because much of this is already overlapping and interrelated. Employing one billing person that can also handle accounts payable and receivable and assist with the monthly profit and loss and general ledger duties is not unheard of while the practice is in the early stages.

A competent and friendly receptionist/phone operator goes a long way.

When a patient walks in to your office, his or her first encounter and impression is made by your receptionist. It is in your best interest to make it a memorable encounter for all the right reasons—not the wrong ones. Rude, dismissive, or incompetent reception area staff will leave your patients with a bad impression of you, despite your best efforts to reverse an unfortunate beginning.

Make sure your phone operator has a pleasant voice, and a friendly personality, and that your patients calling in actually get answers to their questions without making multiple contacts with your office. Basic phone etiquette is not a given, so it is not a bad idea to call the office yourself every so often to make sure that the phone operator is always representing you in a positive light.

Do not let phone calls go unanswered! A missed call is a missed potential patient or referral.

Make sure that someone is always available to take calls and return messages promptly. You never want patients to slip thought the cracks potentially tarnishing your reputation as an attentive physician, and a lost referral will never come back to you. Employ the service of a good answering service for after-hours calls, and make sure they are handling your patient calls competently and courteously. It makes a difference in the eyes of your patients to be treated promptly and respectfully, even in the middle of the night.

Do not let insurance companies play games with your claims!

The insurance companies are in the business of minimizing their costs. Do not be a victim of savvy insurance company personnel trying to deny valid claims, underpaying claims, or trying to bundle procedures. If you are not paying attention, it will cost you.

Make sure your insurance coordinator understands the procedures, files claims in a timely manner, and follows up with claims until they are settled. A little diligence in this area goes a long way.

Consultants

Running a business and caring for patients is a daunting task for even the most organized and energetic physicians, and sometimes the best course of action is to rely on trusted advisors to help in these endeavors. It just makes sense to ask professionals for help in order to minimize costly mistakes in both setting up and running your medical practice.

A good attorney can be a huge asset in good times and in bad.

An attorney will be able to advise you on how to legally structure your business (C-Corp vs. LLC), review and write contracts for you, and render opinions as to whether or not your business practices are in violation of any laws. A trustworthy attorney can set your mind at ease and cut through legalese that you will inevitably encounter dealing with hospital contracts, vendor contracts, and any related business dealings. If you are joining an established practice, it is always a good idea to have your own attorney review your contract for employment to make sure your best interests are addressed. A relationship with an attorney is best fostered from the beginning of your medical practice. The appropriate time to look for an attorney that you trust is never when you *need* one.

A great accountant can be worth their weight in gold.

An accountant will be able to maintain or review your monthly profit and loss statements; file payroll, business, and personal taxes; and most importantly, advise you on how to be the most tax efficient. Taxes are a complex entity, and the correct handling of them from the beginning will save you time and money and maybe even an audit.

A financial planner can help you and your employees plan for the future.

At some point in the life of your medical practice, a financial planner can help you evaluate if a 401k or profit-sharing plan will be beneficial for you and your employees. Understanding the nuances of these plans can help you make the best decisions for you and your staff.

Office Policies

The clearer your office policies are to your staff, the easier their jobs—and yours— will be. Leaving things open to interpretation will only cause undue strife when the inevitable wrong decision is made by an employee, and you have to find a way to "fix" it. Your staff, no matter how competent, needs to know how you would like them to handle specific situations. Top-down management is much clearer than bottom-up.

A comprehensive employee handbook will make everyone's life easier if it is well presented and enforced. You can come up with a handbook with the help of your office manager, and update it as needed in order to guide your employees with the execution of their daily duties. This way, nothing falls through the cracks, and everyone handles things in a uniform manner.

Some areas to consider when drawing up a procedural handbook include:
Patient interaction

- *How will you handle collection of co-pays?*

  - Collection of co-pays at the time of service is advised. It is harder and more expensive to collect these fees after the fact.

- *How will you handle late patients and no-shows?*

  - Will you ask them to reschedule, or will you try to work them in to your schedule?
  - Will you charge no-shows for the missed appointment?
  - Will you discharge chronic no-show patients from your practice if they miss a certain number of appointments?
  - Will you provide appointment reminders or phone calls to minimize no-show rate?

- *What is your billing practice?*

  - Will you provide financial counseling before surgery so that your patient understands the amount that they will pay out-of-pocket to perform the surgery?
  - Will you require your patient to pay all, some, or none of their out-of-pocket expense prior to surgery?
  - The patient's ability to pay should never impact your recommendations, but if the surgery is elective, delaying the surgery in order to collect some or all of the out-of-pocket expense is an option to consider.

- *Will you offer structured repayment plans?*

  - When necessary, structured repayment plans that are comfortable for your patients may be an option.
  - Do not cause your patients financial hardship in order to pay off their debt in 3 months. If they can only afford $5.00 per month, then so be it.

- *How will you handle bad debt?*

  - Will you send patients to a collection service?
  - How many calls will you make to attempt a collection before turning them over to a service?

- *How will you provide results from labs, radiology, or pathology?*

  - Will you call patients personally, or will your nurse deliver results?
  - Will you call only adverse or abnormal results and your nurse deliver normal results?

General office policies

- *How will you handle employee absences, both excused and unexcused?*
- *Will there be a specified dress code, or will your employees be required to purchase and wear scrubs or uniforms?*
- *What are the expectations for conduct and professional courtesy in your office, and what are the repercussions for violating this code of conduct?*
- *Will there be annual reviews for employees, and what is expected of each employee to attain a positive review?*
- *What is the policy for dismissal and written reprimands in your office?*
- *What are the office safety and privacy policies, and how will they be enforced?*

Chapter 29
Building a Program

Adair De Berry-Carlisle and Marc Neff

Introduction

One of the most challenging and rewarding experiences as a surgeon is that of building a program. Whether it is a breast cancer program, or a bariatric program, or a surgical intensivist program, creating something from nothing is an achievement. A new program at your hospital improves patient care, improves your hospital's reputation, is great marketing of your brand, demonstrates your leadership abilities, and creates a legacy for your name. It can also serve to help recruit additional talent in the form of staff and/or surgeons. It can even be a stepping stone to leadership positions in your hospital's organization. It will also be, most likely, a test of your endurance.

Planning

Before you can start building a program, you need to have some serious planning sessions. First off, set your goals. Figure out what you want to achieve. Create a timeline. Figure out the cast of characters. Who do you expect to help you in administration? Where are the finances coming from? What finances are going to be necessary? For example, if I want an accredited bariatric program over the next 5 years, I will need a nursing coordinator, a dietician, a data collector, and a secretary at a minimum. I'm going to need another surgeon for support and an administrator to

A. De Berry-Carlisle, DO, FACOS, FACS (✉)
Trauma and Acute Care Surgery, Surgical Critical Care, St. David's South Austin Medical Center, Austin, TX, USA
e-mail: adeberrycarlisle@yahoo.com

M. Neff, MD, FACS, FASMBS
Center for Surgical Weight Loss, Jefferson Health New Jersey, Cherry Hill, NJ, USA

© Springer International Publishing AG, part of Springer Nature 2018
K. Yoon-Flannery et al. (eds.), *A Surgeon's Path*,
https://doi.org/10.1007/978-3-319-78846-3_29

navigate the hospital committees. I will need to determine a budget for new equipment in the OR and on the hospital floors. I will also need support in the ICU and from radiology. Do this exercise several times. Figure out when you need the support from which characters in your story line.

Once you have figured out the characters and your timeline, start to pitch the idea to others. Be positive. Be engaged. Do the PowerPoint presentations for administration, for nurses, and for fellow surgeons. Expect setbacks. Not everyone will be supportive. There will be the naysayers. People who say it can't be done and will be too expensive to do, that we can't do it as well as a local competitor, and that this isn't what our strategic goal is or should be. This process takes time. When we started building a bariatric program at our hospital, planning took 2 years before we did the first case. Meetings start as small one-on-one or two-on-one. Then gradually expanded to meetings of 15–20 people. We identified an OR team, took them to two different hospitals, practiced the operation four times, and role-played what could go wrong. That degree of strategic planning is necessary if you want your program to be a success.

Along the way, you are going to learn to be a leader. Successful leaders have a defined vision. They have their own personal mission statement. They inspire. They never lose their optimism. They learn to delegate and supervise performance. They build a strong team and they get their buy-in. Be confident. Be detail oriented. Show how the project will be profitable to those involved, the patients, and the hospital as an organization.

Leadership Role

A great idea can quickly become last week's lunch topic if there is no one to fuel momentum. To quote Ben Horowitz, "leaders are neither born nor made; they are found." The goal is to find someone who can infuse others with their passion. In order to build any program or organization, someone, somewhere, starts with a passion for a cause. In our profession, this is the easy part. Our cause is to improve care and quality of life. So many in the medical profession have wonderful, grand ideas to this end. The hard part is herding the cats in one direction. Confidence is seldom lacking but the ability to lead is a rare gem. The great leaders are not always the high profile and big personalities. In fact, they are often quiet if not shy. One thing they all have in common is their ability to put together the right team, getting the right people in and the wrong people out.

Whatever we do in our capacity as medical professionals is centered around one guiding principle: the patient comes first—they *always* come first. A successful leader not only embraces this concept but also has the ability to articulate their vision to others. The team will continue the momentum created by the leader. The number one cause of team disruption is lack of communication. A strong leader knows their team: their strengths and weaknesses. When working with a team, you can focus on one of two paths: personality or behavior. You will never change an individual's personality but you can change their behavior, so choose wisely.

Successful teams move in the same direction. Meetings can quickly deteriorate into arguments based on differing points of view. An alternative is to discuss ideas along the lines of strategic thinking. For example, what is beneficial about the idea, what is potentially problematic, what emotions does it evoke, is there a creative alternative, and of course, is this financially responsible? Productive decisions can then be made when all avenues have been discussed.

Do not waiver and remember the big picture. The accomplishments of the program are what matter. This is the purpose of your endeavor. Be confident in your goals and be able to say without reservation that what you are doing is right. Be supportive of your team. Be quick to complement and give credit. This is a labor of love that requires self-sacrifice and humility. Push people to be their best through leading by example not force. Kindness and strength are not mutually exclusive and when intertwined will produce a lasting success.

Along the way, don't be frustrated by setbacks. You may not get the support staff or equipment you feel you need in the next budget cycle. Don't give up. You may have an early complication in patient care. You may find that you are losing you zeal for the project. Don't give up. When you are tired, learn to take a break and remember it is ok to ask for help. It is very hard when you are trying to be a busy and productive surgeon and have a life outside of the hospital, to find the time to build something brand new. Take just a few minutes each and every day and the time and effort will start adding up. As a final reminder, it is easy to get distracted from the goal along the way. Whatever your program may be, from starting a training program to redefining trauma excellence, just remember who you are ultimately doing this for the patient.

Chapter 30
Lawsuits

Marc Neff

Introduction

Disclaimer, I am not a lawyer. I have never wanted to be one. I was married to a lawyer and have several good friends who are lawyers. But after five malpractice suits, one complicated divorce, multiple contract reviews, and one civil suit a patient brought against me, I've sadly met enough lawyers in my medical career to be able to write this chapter. I'm going to focus here on *malpractice cases*.

Malpractice Cases

First comment, an ounce of prevention is worth the investment. Be honest with your patients and their families and in your documentation in the chart. It is well known that just because you make a mistake or an error is perceived, it doesn't mean you are going to get sued. People sue because they feel you wronged them and didn't own up to it or that you tried to hide it. They sue because they think you didn't care that you made a mistake and that the mistakes kept happening and because they weren't involved in the decision-making process. The majority of patients understand that you aren't perfect. They expect, though, that you can get them out of whatever trouble they are in, and that's why they went to someone who completed 28th grade before they started practicing medicine. Be explicit in the chart; it is a legal document. It will be the evidence used in 2–3 years when this eventually comes to the point of depositions. What you were thinking, why you did what you did, what really happened, what you told the patient and the family, and what they understood all will be there in the chart.

M. Neff, MD, FACS, FASMBS
Center for Surgical Weight Loss, Jefferson Health New Jersey, Cherry Hill, NJ, USA

© Springer International Publishing AG, part of Springer Nature 2018
K. Yoon-Flannery et al. (eds.), *A Surgeon's Path*,
https://doi.org/10.1007/978-3-319-78846-3_30

Second comment, it sucks. We went into this career to help people, not to hurt them. We, however, are not perfect. Even if you are 99% perfect and you do more than a hundred cases a year, you are going to hurt one person. If you are 99.9% perfect, you are going to hurt 1 in a 1000. The average general surgeon will do 400–500 cases a year and over 15,000 in a 30-year career. You are going to make some mistakes, some days when you were distracted, and some days when you were not at your best. Those days won't typically be your worst days ever; they will just be when you lost focus.

So, you commit an error. What are the first things to do? Well, first off, discuss it with your partners. Their names will be on the chart somewhere. Even if they don't get drawn into it, they may need to cover for you during your depositions/trial, so don't be afraid to reach out for their help and advice. And listen to it. They've likely been there. And, generally, they want what's best for you. Second, notify your malpractice carrier. They want to know as early as possible what's going on. Let them start building a chart. This shows them you are honest and forthright. They, after all, are going to be paid to defend you. Third, there is likely a risk management officer at the hospital. They, and/or the chief of surgery, need to know what is going on. Just as with your partners, the hospital may be drawn into whatever may happen down the road. It is best to be honest and upfront (a repeated theme here). While every institution is different, many times the individuals listed above can help navigate disclosure of the error with the patient and the family. Most of the time, physicians are encouraged to be honest about mistakes but, especially in the beginning, seek guidance in how best to disclose this information.

Ok, so, you've committed an error and believe it's likely to be a malpractice case. Now what? First, continue with appropriate medical care for the patient. Do everything to the letter of the textbook. Also, be honest when you are in over your head. Don't try repairing a bile duct that you severed if you've never done it before. Make sure documentation is perfect too. Read everything, from labs to consults to diagnostic studies. Speak with everyone, resident, nurse, consulting physician, and whoever sees or touches the patient. With the first error, patients can maybe forgive, but not the second one, and errors tend to beget more errors.

Even if you do all of these things but believe that a malpractice suit is inevitable, remember that you still have 300 more patients this year and 500 next year that need your entire focus. It will be hard and distracting to read letters from the malpractice carrier and meeting with the lawyers, but you still need to be present and mindful of what you are doing day in and day out. And that regards what happens out of the hospital too. You may have a partner, a spouse, children, parents, or other family members that depend on you too, and you can't go around sulking that you pitched a bad game and lost it for the team. You have a job to do. Being a professional means keeping your mind-set on the present.

The meeting with the lawyer is the first step. After many letters have gone back and forth, you will meet with your attorney. He/she will want to know what happened during the case. They will want you to explain to them the medical side. Be honest and upfront. What you did right and what you did wrong. What you could have done better. What you said to the patient and the family. They will want to review parts of the chart with you including operative notes and consultant reports. Remember, they are on your side. Bare your soul to them. They are assessing you as a witness, the case as a whole. Is it defensible? Should we settle? They have experience with similar cases and have interviewed many, many doctors. Give them the credit they deserve and remember that they are on your side. What's going through their mind is, if 100 surgeons were in your position, what would the majority of them have done? Medicine is not an exact science. The courts know that. But the standard of care is what the majority would do, and that's the measure you are up against.

Experts

What a crazy name. I've never felt comfortable with the idea of an expert. I've been out for over 15 years, done over 1300 weight loss surgeries; does that make me an expert? Someone who testifies well, has an impressive CV, and may want the extra cash; they can be the experts. Your case might come down to how your expert fairs compared to theirs. I've been in a case where the expert had less experience than me, but came off better than our expert, and sadly, I ended up losing that case. You want your expert to be an expert in every sense of the word. What they write about your case, how they speak and explain things, their list of credentials, and even their presence/charisma. Your attorney may ask you for suggestions. Big names are good here, and you can ask around, but they often have a list of potential experts. The expert will first review your case and write a summary for the attorney. Read it carefully. Be honest if you think they aren't going to be good for the case. An up-to-date literature review related to your case may be helpful as well to share with your counsel. Your attorney will then render an opinion. Listen to it. If they think it's time to settle, don't argue. It's in the expert's best interests to appear in court, they make more money that way, but if they don't think it's defensible at the point of the initial case review, it's time to lick your wounds and move on.

Depositions

Truly a horrible process, worse than board exams. You go into a room with your lawyer, the opposing lawyer, a big pile of documents, and a court recorder. You swear an oath, and then you answer questions until the opposing council is done. My quickest was 1.5 h, and the opposing lawyer yelled at me several times, "What did you do wrong?" The process could take more than 1 day. Remember, this is just about the facts. Stick to them. Pause before you answer any question. Don't give in to emotion. Ask for clarification if you don't understand. Don't guess. Don't get involved in "what ifs" and hypotheticals. Hopefully, your attorney will give you this advice as well and review with you. Give your attorney an opportunity to object to a question if they don't like how it was asked. You can take a break if you need to (it's wise to do so after 2 h just to breathe and go to the bathroom). Don't volunteer anything. It's the plaintiff's attorney's job to get the information they want. Just answer what was asked and stop there. A "where did you go to medical school question" needs only to be answered by the name of the medical school, not a listing of the awards you received while you were there or that you took a year off to do research in the lab.

What if I'm named with my partner/colleague? This is a tough one. I can only give you my personal experience here. First of all, you are both in this together, so it doesn't do any good to fight over who had more to do with what happened to the patient or to play the blame game. You have to keep working with your partner and even figure out how to cover each other during the process of depositions/trial. Secondly, your partner is going through the same tough time you are with the case. Emotionally, these cases take a toll (addressed below), and they likely have some raw nerves related to the case as well. Here's where you need to discuss things with your malpractice carrier and your attorney privately. You may have a meeting that includes your partner, but their job is to defend you. If you don't feel like you are getting adequate representation, speak up now, or forever hold your peace. You can't wait until the case is over to think to yourself that I should have had separate counsel.

Will this take a toll on your health? Definitely. From the beginning of this chapter, when I said it "sucked," to the parts where you have to list this case on all of your applications for credentialing, to the next time you are faced with such a complicated case to perform, to answering your family's questions about how it went. Your stress level is going to be high. A malpractice case is like a noose around your neck until it's completed, and they don't go away quickly, and they can overlap with other malpractice cases at the same time. There is no limit that says this surgeon has enough on their plate right now, and we can wait until the time is right to bring this suit up (actually, the statute is 2 years from the date of recognized injury). Not to be dismissive, but it's somewhat the cost of doing business. The average general surgeon gets sued once every 5 years (sadly, I'm a little better than average). You can't let a malpractice case destroy everything you've worked your entire life to accomplish and achieve. Remember to eat well and that exercise is a great way to burn off steam, and don't keep emotions bottled up inside. Talk to your spouse; don't take out your frustration on them or your kids. The information you share with your spouse is privileged and protected and can't be used against you. They are your partners in life, through good times and bad, so use them. If you are with a good one, they will be focused on what you are going through and how they can help you, and not how it's going to impact them or your future bill-paying ability. Finally, some large hospitals or academic centers may have assistance for dealing with the emotional toll of going through a lawsuit. If you have a risk management office, they may be able to guide you here.

One last comment, regardless of how bad you feel or how much you are trying to right a wrong, don't give patients or family members your cell phone number. Been there, done that. It can be used against you, and there is no break for you if you are answering questions night and day. In one of my cases, 17 pages of text messages were submitted as evidence. You will do it someday and learn it's a gesture that has no meaning or value and only robs you of what little sanity you will have left.

Part IV
After Starting Your First Job

Chapter 31
Preparing for Your First Day on the Job

Linda Szczurek

Think back about 5–6 years ago and remember your first day as an intern. If you are like the most of us, one Friday you were a fourth year medical student and the following Monday you were a doctor. This title came with a lot more responsibility, and you were probably very nervous and unsure of yourself. Welcome to your first day as an attending; it will be a hundred times worse. You are now completely responsible for everything that happens to your patients. I can guarantee that you will be anxious and constantly questioning yourself when you first start. The good news is that this feeling is totally normal!

The first few days at your new job will likely involve orientation with a ton of paperwork, computer training, and introductions to a lot of new people. A lot of this paperwork will occur prior to your start date. Usually, a hospital or private practice will not let you start until you have filled out all of the paperwork for credentialing ahead of time. You will need to submit copies of the following: driver's license, social security card, diplomas from college and medical school, graduation certificates from internship/residency/fellowship, state medical license, US Drug Enforcement Administration (DEA) license, Controlled Dangerous Substance (CDS) registration, letters of recommendation, as well as other items such as case logs. There will be human resources paperwork to fill out for health insurance, retirement accounts, and other benefits that your job includes.

Hospitals have credentialing committees, and all of your paperwork needs to be complete prior to privilege approval before you can start working. The hospital will provide you with a list of all the different types of surgical procedures, and you will have to request any or all the cases that you plan to do. In some cases, for advanced procedures and procedures that require certain equipment or skills, the hospital may actually ask to see documentation that you have been properly trained. Finally, you will be required to complete/sign credentialing paperwork to be enrolled in all of the

L. Szczurek, DO, FACOS
Jefferson Health New Jersey, Cherry Hill, NJ, USA

© Springer International Publishing AG, part of Springer Nature 2018
K. Yoon-Flannery et al. (eds.), *A Surgeon's Path*,
https://doi.org/10.1007/978-3-319-78846-3_31

different insurance panels. Most institutions will not let you start working until you are approved by many of the insurance panels for billing reasons.

The remainder of the orientation and computer training are very similar to the previous experience you went through as an intern, resident, and/or fellow. This will include going over hospital policies, taking a tour of the facility, and obtaining an ID badge and access to the areas of the building where you will be working. Hopefully, the hospital has a user-friendly electronic health record (EHR) or one that you are familiar with; otherwise your first few working days may be a struggle as you learn the new system. If you are working as an employee for one hospital system, this orientation process should not take too long. However, if you are working for a private practice and/or will have privileges at more than one hospital system, you may be in for a lot more work and time. Different hospital systems will likely have different credentialing processes and possibly different EHR systems.

The most important part of the orientation process will be meeting the administrators, other physicians, and staff at the hospital. Everyone knows how important first impressions are, and you want to make a great one! This means that you should be well rested and ready to go the first day of work. You should be well dressed and groomed. No, you cannot roll out of bed and throw on scrubs to show up on day one at your new job even if you are a surgeon. You should be wearing suitable business attire and make sure that you have your white coat and ID badge with you. Make it a point to be kind and courteous and introduce yourself to everyone that you meet. You will be meeting many new people in a very short period of time. Remembering people's names will go a long way. You can also ask for their business cards or contact information for future use.

Keeping on the topic of good impressions, there is a very fine line between confidence and arrogance. I learned something very important from playing sports in college in a program founded on tradition; we refer to it as "quiet confidence." This means that as an attending, you convey to your new colleagues and patients that you *are* smart, hardworking, and trustworthy, a leader, and good at what you were trained to do by both your words and actions. This does not mean that you think you know everything, do not take the time to listen to others, or think that you know more than your new colleagues and patients. The wrong attitude will follow you through your career if you are not careful. If you treat everyone well from the beginning, they will enjoy working with you and you with them.

Do not be afraid to ask a lot of questions. Where do I park? How do I get scrubs and a locker? What is the process for booking an emergency case? Who do I call if there is a problem with _____? What time is the cafeteria open? You will learn the answers to most of your questions on the fly, but if you can think of them ahead of time, it will be much easier to be prepared ahead of time rather than trying to figure out the answers later.

You may find yourself in situations that are completely foreign to you and will need help in the beginning. The best example that I can provide is billing. Residents and fellows have little exposure to medical billing during training, but this will now become very important as this is how you are paid. Your partners will be able to quickly teach you a few billing basics to help you get started. For more in depth information, try contacting one of the billing specialists at the hospital or in your new office. In addition, there are many resources online and billing courses that you can take. If you are not at all familiar with the basic billing and procedure codes, you should do a little research on the topic prior to your first day at work or sign up for a quick class during your time off between completing training and starting your new job. *Never* be afraid or too proud to ask for help no matter what the situation.

Prior to your first case in your new hospital/operating room, you should make some time to specifically meet with the OR nurse manager and the person responsible for equipment. You will need to help make your preference cards. These are lists of all the supplies that you will need for different cases. Having these items ahead of time will ensure that your surgeries go much smoother and on time. The OR staff will want to know exactly which items you want opened at the beginning of the case and which items you would like them to have on hold in the room in case you need the item at some point. If you spent all of your training at one institution, you may be very familiar with certain OR equipment, but not all hospitals have the same supplies. If your new OR does not have what you are used to working with, they will likely have a substitute. At the main hospital where I work, we have Monocryl suture for closing skin. The first time I went to one of the other hospitals, I learned they did not carry Monocryl. Good thing the OR staff is usually helpful and told me that they use Biosyn suture which is an equivalent. There may be a product that you absolutely need that your new OR does not carry, and you will need to find out if they will be able to order the product for you. Some of the other equipment such as the laparoscopic cameras, vessel sealant devices, and bowel staplers may also not be the same brands that you are accustomed to using. I recommend that you speak with the staff and any of the product representatives before your first case so that you are familiar with the products and equipment available before using it for the first time.

A few other quick tips that will be helpful include: Make sure that you pack some healthy snacks and or lunch. Many hospitals have a doctor's lounge that will have coffee, water, and some snacks to munch on, but these are often not very healthy options. Some smaller hospitals may have times when the cafeteria is closed, and you don't want to miss lunch time and have to go all day without eating or order unhealthy take out frequently. Do not forget to bring OR shoes to leave in you scrub locker. Dress shoes are uncomfortable to stand in for a long case, and we all know that the shoe covers are permeable to liquids which can lead to many ruined shoes and socks. If you are relocating and are not too familiar with the area, you may want to map out the quickest ways to get around. This will help with your time management especially on busy days.

Lastly, you may have at least a few days between the end of your training and your official start date. You should certainly take advantage of these days to relax and enjoy yourself; read a good book, go on vacation, or spend time with family. This may be the one opportunity where you can take a few days off without really having to worry about work-related things. And if you have the luxury of taking extra time off, I highly suggest taking advantage to the opportunity.

Chapter 32
Dealing with Your Clinic

Linda Szczurek and Nicole M. Saur

Introduction

Every surgeon likes to do things slightly differently. Starting a new job as an attending will give you the opportunity to organize your clinic/office hours the way you like. Chances are you will be joining an already established group or a hospital-based practice. The office may already function like a well-oiled machine, but if not, this allows you the chance to step in with some fresh new ideas on how to organize the office to function more smoothly and improve patient care and satisfaction.

Questions to Ask

Prior to your first day in clinic/office hours, we recommend that you sit down with the office manager and any of the other staff that you will work with on a daily basis (surgery scheduler, medical assistant, front desk, and billing) and at least one of your new partners. You want to get a good idea of how the office currently runs.

How are the appointments scheduled: What time are the office hours? How long are patient appointments? Do they take into consideration new patient appointments versus postoperative appointments which are usually much shorter? Are there procedure appointments? If you are not available, will your partners cover your patients for office visits? If a patient does not show up for their appointment, does the office staff call to reschedule?

L. Szczurek, DO, FACOS (✉)
Jefferson Health New Jersey, Cherry Hill, NJ, USA

N. M. Saur, MD
Division of Colon and Rectal Surgery, Department of Surgery,
University of Pennsylvania, Philadelphia, PA, USA

© Springer International Publishing AG, part of Springer Nature 2018
K. Yoon-Flannery et al. (eds.), *A Surgeon's Path*,
https://doi.org/10.1007/978-3-319-78846-3_32

What equipment/supplies do they have in the office: Do the current members of the group do any office procedures? Do they have the supplies that you normally use for dressing changes or any procedures that you plan on doing in the office? If you need to order new equipment or supplies, it is typically easier if you ask for them before starting your clinic. If you have equipment you can't live without, particularly if it is expensive, this can even be negotiated as part of your contract (e.g., in colon and rectal surgery, proctology tables, flexible sigmoidoscopes, etc.).

What is the current patient flow in the office: What is the role of each staff member? What is the responsibility of the medical assistant (rooming patients, vitals, entry into the electronic medical record (EMR), chart prep, assisting with office procedures, making sure the patient rooms have all the necessary supplies)? What is the current method for scheduling patients for surgery? Do you have to fill out any of the scheduling paperwork and give slips for preadmission testing or does the staff do these things? If you want to order a test that requires precertification such as a CT or MRI, who is responsible for this? Who answers patient phone calls? Do you have an advanced practice provider (nurse practitioner, physician's assistant, etc.) working with you in the office?

Staffing

Especially as a new attending, it is very valuable to have another practitioner helping with office hours, phone calls, and preoperative preparation of your patients. I recommend determining if one is available to you before you start working, and, if not, I would again recommend negotiating this into your contract, if possible. What is the procedure for following up with patients to make sure the test gets done and you get the results? How does billing work? Do you have to put the correct billing/CPT codes on office notes (don't forget about daily hospital rounds and surgery)?

Once you find out the answers to these questions, you will be able to decide what works well for you and what you would like to change in order to make your day run more efficiently. If there are significant changes that you would like to make, you should sit down with the office manager and review these changes. If these changes will affect any of your new partners, you should also speak with them to get their opinion. Who knows? They may have tried your idea already, and for some reason it did not work.

Schedule

The best and easiest change that the office will likely be able to accommodate is your office schedule. You will need to give your staff an idea of how long you will need to spend with different types of patients. You do not want the staff giving a patient with a newly diagnosed cancer a 15 min appointment because they will have many questions and concerns. Once you start to get behind in office hours, it is very hard to catch up. The same will apply to office procedures if you plan on doing these in the office. In contrast, you do not want them scheduling a quick post-op visit for 30 min when it will take 10 min. It may also take you some time to get used to completing your charts in the EMR as this is much more time consuming than hand writing a quick note.

When you first start, you should review the details of your day and scheduling with the office staff. You want to make sure they give you adequate time for things such as travel to and from places; i.e., if you have OR scheduled in the morning and office hours in the afternoon, you want to make sure you will not be rushing through the OR cases or worse running late to office hours. You will already feel overwhelmed, and the last thing you need is a waiting room of angry patients. You should also consider if you would be willing to see add-on patients the same day. It's ok if you are not very busy, but if the office already has you overbooked, this can start to cause issues. Do you get a formal lunch break? Or do you wind up seeing patients straight through until the afternoon? This decision is totally up to you, but it is nice to be able to sit down for a few minutes in the middle of the day. Trust me; you will have other things you can catch up on during this time such as your EMR, patient phone calls, and signing off on other paperwork.

Chart Preparation

Another important item that can keep you on schedule or slow you down is chart preparation. You want to make sure that your office staff has collected all of the items that the patient will need prior to their appointment. This means that if a new patient is coming to see you and has imaging studies, labs, etc., which were already done by the referring physician, the patient should be asked to bring all of these to the office for their appointment. In addition, it is even more helpful if your staff can find out where the testing was done and already have a copy of the reports in the patients chart for you to review before walking in the room to see the patient. When these steps are not followed, the office staff will usually try to call the lab, imaging facility, or other doctor's office to get this information, but it often requires more paperwork in terms of medical release forms and can take time. You will not want to waste time waiting for the results, and the patient does not want to sit and wait for you until the results arrive. The chart preparation also applies to postoperative patient information as you will want copies of the operative report and any pathology results available for the appointment. Preparation ahead of time also works well for procedures. If you or your staff knows that a patient is coming to the office for a procedure, it will help keep you organized and on time if the staff has the room set up ahead of time. This will include having any consent forms that the patient will need to sign available, any typed instructions that you would like to give the patient after the procedure, and equipment and dressings that you will require.

Documentation

The most time-consuming element of office hours will be your documentation in the electronic medical record. Some doctors find it difficult to type on the computer and talk to the patient at the same time, and some patients feel the doctor is not listening to them if their head is behind a monitor typing away. Fortunately, EMR is now so common that most patients have gotten used to this way of practice. We do recommend that you try as hard as you can to complete most of your charts during office hours or right after. It is very easy to get behind when you are trying to see 15–20 patients in a morning or afternoon. If you do not finish the chart work during hours, you will wind up with what we refer to as "surgery homework." You will already be working long days, and the last thing you will want to do is spend 2 hours at night or on the weekend completing leftover charts. Furthermore, when you do not complete your charts during the office visit or shortly after, it is difficult to remember all of the details that you need to put into your notes, and patient's information will blend together. Failure to complete your charts in a timely fashion can also affect surgery scheduling because the history and physical will be needed for the day of the surgery.

Procedures

A quick word on office procedures—most new surgery attendings starting their first job out of residency or fellowship will not have a vast knowledge of office procedures unless you had a dedicated rotation during your residency. Before doing any office procedures, you really need to make sure that your staff is trained in how to assist with procedures and that you have all of the supplies and equipment that you will need. If the staff does not know exactly what to do and you don't have everything in the procedure room, this will not turn out well. Remember, these patients are completely awake and will remember exactly what happened and what was said. If the patient is not completely confident in your skills and the procedure does not go smoothly, they will look for another surgeon next time they need something. Our best advice with this is to start small, like an excision of a small skin lesion in an easily accessible location or drainage of an abscess. You should be aware that you will probably not have the same bright lighting and electrocautery that you are used to in the OR. Make sure that you get a full history from the patient prior to the procedure specifically if they are taking any anticoagulants. Once you are comfortable with the smaller procedures and know that your staff is well trained and you have all the equipment, you can try to do more advanced procedures in the office such as excision of a small soft tissue mass or scalp wen. We will caution you with two points: (1) Back skin is much thicker than it looks, and those small appearing sebaceous cysts often go down to the muscle layer. (2) The head/neck/scalp has a very profuse blood supply. It will take some time for you to become comfortable doing some procedures in the office. As a rule of thumb, if you have any doubt that you can't do the procedure in the office, then be smart and safe and schedule it for the OR.

Communication with Staff

One of the easiest things that you can do to make your day run smoothly is to be nice to *all* of your staff. This means no yelling and barking orders at them when you are having a bad day. Be assured that this will not work in any situation including the office or the OR. This only makes everyone including the patients frustrated. If one of the staff is not doing their job correctly or making the same mistake on a regular basis, you should correct them by explaining the issue and how to correct it. If this becomes a consistent problem, it should be relayed to the office manager to handle. Joining a practice that has been established for some time, there is a high probability that the office staff have also been working there and together for a long time. You may start to pick up on the staff/staff and staff/physician relationships. Try to stay out of any drama that may occur throughout the office.

Final Thoughts

Many surgeons dread office hours because they would rather spend more time operating. You need to remember that office hours will be a vital part of most surgeons' practices. Office hours are where you will schedule most of your cases. When you start your hours off in a good mindset and with proper organization, they can run smoothly and stress free for everyone.

Chapter 33
Navigating Electronic Medical Records

Robert Neff and Jonathan Nguyen

Definition and Disambiguation

Before we begin talking about EMRs, let's spend the time to define and call out some common three-letter acronyms, which often get confused.

EHRs are electronic health records.

EMRs are electronic medical records.

PHRs are (electronic) personal health records.

The Office of the National Coordinator for Healthcare Technology (ONC) [1] defines EHRs and EMRs separately—however these terms are often used interchangeably.

"An EMR contains the standard medical and clinical data gathered in one provider's office. Electronic health records (EHRs) go beyond the data collected in the provider's office and include a more comprehensive patient history."

Electronic personal health records, however, are different, and they are not in very common use. The best way of thinking of a PHR is as an EMR that the patient is in control of. There were several large tech companies which started experimenting with this technology around the year 2010. These included Microsoft (Microsoft HealthVault), Google (Google Health), and many startups that were focused solely on these types of systems. While many of these tools were great solutions, they were searching for a problem. The hope that patients would become engaged in their

R. Neff, BSc (✉)
Digital Innovation and Consumer Experience Group (DICE),
Thomas Jefferson University and Jefferson Health,
Philadelphia, PA, USA
e-mail: robert.neff@jefferson.edu

J. Nguyen, DO
Division of Trauma and Critical Care,
Morehouse School of Medicine,
Atlanta, GA, USA

health to the extent that they would manage their own records was ahead of its time (and still is a little bit ahead today). Additionally, the challenge for patients to share data stored in these PHR systems with their providers proved formidable.

In addition to these clinical systems, it is critical to realize that in any health system, or even small practice, the EMR/EHR is a critical clinical system, but it is not the only software system (or even the only clinical software system). There are other systems that manage everything from human resources (employment and pay-checks) to medical devices, to the Internet/websites, to phone systems, and more. There are also mobile apps which might or might not be part of the clinical system. These will be further discussed in the section of this chapter on interoperability—however it's important to understand that while the EMR might be the primary system that a provider uses, it is only one of several systems which the patient and other staff use.

This chapter will focus on EMRs and EHRs, and their use in the inpatient (acute care), outpatient (ambulatory), and, to a small extent, population health systems.

History of EMRs

The first electronic medical records were created as databases to electronically store data that was previously written on paper. There are numerous benefits to an electronic approach, as one can imagine. These initial benefits included the ability to have backups of the information, allowing better searching for data and sharing across a single health system—and perhaps most importantly for some, to give a method to quickly and accurately handle the medical billing.

As technology improved and new features were added, physician workflows were added to the system. These workflows made it possible to collect data in the same way and standardize care across providers. Of course, this came with challenges to the providers—but it allowed for a more unified experience for the patients. It also allowed for systems to be built to aid the provider in his or her care. For example, systems were soon able to check for medication conflicts and prevent potentially serious and life-threatening interactions.

As the EMR became more and more integral in the care and the workflow of the provider—features were added to these systems to do much more than simply record patients' health conditions and bill insurance companies for the care. The systems began to manage operational aspects of the health system. Almost any operational activity that occurs in the hospital is now offered in some sense in the EMR, because each of these activities creates data that must end up in the EMR.

Today, most EMRs have modules to register patients, manage their movement throughout the hospital, send prescriptions to pharmacies, view imaging results, send messages to providers, and manage the dispensing of medication through bar code medication administration (BCMA).

Principles and Methods Behind EHRs

As they are now, EHRs provide physicians an unparalleled advantage in the care of our patients. From anywhere in the world, they can quickly access their medication lists, labs, imaging, consultation notes, and more. It eliminates the situation in which multiple providers are trying to access and document on the same chart at once. Multiple users can simultaneously write notes, review orders, and trend vitals and outputs without hindering their colleagues. Having electronic records also helps make paper charts obsolete. The days of sifting through boxes of patient data are over, as this can be easily done with the help of search tools. EHRs can also track patients, alert you to avoid potential medical errors, and even alarm if a patient meets certain criteria. The crux to all this is that EHR is still only a tool. At the end of the day, a tool is only as good as the surgeon's skill in wielding it.

How EHRs Feed Information for Reporting

CMS has set forth a series of objectives that EHR and hospitals must try and hit in order to prove that they are effectively using EHR to gather data and improve quality of care in their institution. This is what's called "meaningful use." The aim of this was to help ensure that providers gathered adequate information on their patients including medications, social history, etc. The second portion of this required that institutions start reporting certain quality measures such as their ability to control blood pressure, heart failure readmissions, iatrogenic pneumothorax, etc. By tracking and trending these core measures, a hospital in theory could identify issues and resolve them.

On an institution-wide level, they are able to use EHR to track your progress as a physician. They can track how long it takes you to see a clinic patient and close out their charts, the number of times you don't order DVT prophylaxis, how fast you sign orders, how many incomplete charts you have, and how long it takes you to do your dictation for cases.

Why Should Doctors Care About Any of This?

The reason this is important is because it can lead to a better financial return back for the hospital. The hospital is judged on how many of the meaningful use criteria are met. If the institution does not make these marks, they may suffer a penalty. The amount of financial incentive is based on the complexity of charts which you can look up at the link https://www.cms.gov/Regulations-and-Guidance/Legislation/EHRIncentivePrograms/index.html?redirect=/ehrincentiveprograms/. On a physician level, many institutions utilize this information for two reasons. If you are not meeting their internal metrics, the powers that be are informed and disciplinary or educations actions may be taken. If your medical records are not up to date, they may suspend your privileges, and there's nothing worse than a surgeon who can't get into the operating room. Some hospitals also withhold a percentage of your paycheck for "quality." This is not a bonus, but a way the hospital gets you to follow their priorities. If your percentages don't line up with their expectations, you don't get that money back. It's important to discuss with your employer about these issues so that you understand how you are being measured and evaluated.

Will EHRs Slow You Down?

The short answer is *yes*. But hopefully only at first. As we mentioned earlier, EHR is only a tool that you have to learn how to use. Regardless of whether you've used the same system before, you'll still need to go through an orientation because each iteration of the same software is different. Pay attention to the differences and be sure to find the contact info for someone in the information technology (IT) department that can help you later on. You'll inevitably need it as you start putting in orders and writing notes. Discuss with others in your group about what note template and order sets they use. Usually there are physician champions who found a way to optimize this already, and you may not need to reinvent the wheel. If you find that you can make one better, talk with IT, and streamline your templates to help you move faster.

How Can You Help Your EHR Be Better?

One of the most interesting things about any EMR system is that if you have seen it in one health system, you have really only seen it at one health system. The same EMR may look and behave differently at each hospital, health system, or practice where it is used. There are hundreds of thousands of permutations on how a system can be configured. This leads to why it is so difficult to implement, interoperate, and support.

During an EMR implementation, experts across the health system are consulted to determine exactly how to configure an EMR to best support the existing and desired workflows of the organization. There are additionally several committees in place throughout every organization whose goal is to continuously refine the way the system is configured to enhance the capabilities (whether that is through new additions to the systems, added features in the EMR, or custom-developed add-ons).

Almost every IT shop in a health system is anxious to work with the providers to improve their experience with the EMR. It is important to look at the IT department as your partner in improving the system. There are often many very frustrating, but valid reasons why a system is set up the way it is. Your best chance of getting the system changed is to understand why it is configured as it is right now. Only then can you figure out how best to optimize the system to meet your needs while not impacting someone else's needs/requirements negatively. Often times for billing, regulatory, or quality reasons, the system is configured in a certain way, and a conversation with those departments may allow adjustments to be made so that everyone's needs can be met.

How Can Data Be Shared Across Systems?

Interoperability is perhaps one of the most frustrating parts of the healthcare industry, particularly as it comes to EMRs. It is hard enough to exchange data between EMRs by the same manufacturer let alone EMRs from different manufacturers.

There are some great standard organizations in place, the most prominent of them the Health Level Seven International (HL7) [2]. Founded in 1987, HL7 is a not-for-profit, American National Standards Institute (ANSI)-accredited organization dedicated to providing a comprehensive framework and related standards for the exchange, integration, sharing, and retrieval of electronic health information that supports clinical practice and the management, delivery, and evaluation of health services.

Despite the great work of groups like HL7, exchange of data across EMRs is very hard. The challenge of the exchange of healthcare data is twofold. The first general problem is one of taxonomy and nomenclature. A given EMR might refer to blood pressure (BP) in many different ways. A patient might have different types of BP such as IVBP, NIBP, and BP and might have several of each of these—taken in different parts of the body. When exchanging this data with another system, it is necessary to map these data elements across—and even two EMRs from the same manufacturer might use these fields differently. The second general problem is one of reconciliation. Most patients have profiles/encounters/records in multiple different EMRs because they have been seen by providers in different organizations. When data from one system is shared with a second, there is a manual step required to reconcile all the conflicting information in each system. An example of this is a patient in EMR-A which is listed as taking atorvastatin (generic) 10 mg and having that record imported into EMR-B which lists the patient taking Lipitor (brand) 20 mg. A provider must review this data and determine (often time in consultation with the patient) what the current state actually is. Did the patient switch to a generic and lower the dose? Is the patient accidentally taking one of each because he or she doesn't realize they are the same? It is important to correct this, in the system—and possibly also in real life. All this reconciliation work takes a lot of time—and this is just a simple case. The EMR cannot (and should not) do it by itself.

Additionally, it is only responsible to note that there are few incentives for EMR manufacturers, and even providers, to make it easy to exchange healthcare information. After all, healthcare is a business, and we would all prefer that our patients get the best care they can but get it from our providers.

Why Is This All So Hard and Complicated?

The concept of EHR seems so simple. Make a computer program that records patient health information and allows us to place orders and review labs and make it universal so the information can be shared. Like many things in medicine, the answer is not so black and white. Every hospital has different priorities, structures, policies, and workflows. Even if the same EHR software is used, the program is tailored to that institution's needs. Add on the fact that every physician specialty and even group can have different priorities and needs that must be considered. Top that all off with every other ancillary service in the hospital that is required to keep the lights on. Each one of these adds another level of complexity to the programming that must grow alongside the hospital's needs.

On a global level, EHRs are also a business. Their goal is to provide a system that does the job the client needs while making a profit. While they are here to help make our lives easier, they have no incentive to make each system interchangeable or standardized.

Whether you like it or not, EHRs are here to stay. As the primary users and caretakers of this information, it is critical that we help shape the way it's used in our hospitals and to mold the way EHR is deployed universally.

References

1. Definition and Benefits of Electronic Medical Records (EMR). The Office of the National Coordinator for Healthcare Technology. Providers & Professionals.
2. Health Level Seven International. http://www.hl7.org/implement/standards/ansiapproved.cfm

Chapter 34
First Call with Your First Emergent Case as an Attending

Linda Szczurek and Holly Graves

It is eventually going to happen. You have completed all of those years of general surgery training, and you are now the attending. Inherent to being a surgeon, you will encounter an emergency. An emergency obviously takes different contexts in the setting of different specialties, but the bottom line is universal—someone needs your help now. The first thing to realize is that you can only do your best as no physician is or will ever be perfect. Remember that you are highly trained and all you can do is give you best effort. The second course of action to take is to remain calm. If you lose your cool, so will the rest of the team, who is relying on you for leadership. Remember how many years you spent in training to prepare for this moment.

So it happens, you are the surgeon on call and you get the call. First, ensure you get a complete history. Remember you may be at home or in the office or even in a different hospital rounding. First question to consider, can the hospital support this case? Any hospital in America can handle an appendectomy, but can your facility properly care for a ruptured abdominal aortic aneurysm or trauma patient? In these extreme circumstances, patients must be transferred to the nearest tertiary care facility. Most hospitals will have contracts and/or relationships with academic centers. However, in other cases you may be asked to facilitate a transfer, so get to know the surgical specialists in your area.

Once you have taken on an emergent case, you need to know how to use your time wisely. If you are at home or the office and driving to the hospital, use your best tool—your phone. Call your resident to perform a prudent physical exam, speak to radiology if you need a stat scan done or a stat read performed, tell the ER or ICU to give the patient fluids or blood or critical medication before the OR, and talk to the OR and tell them what equipment you need. This may be obvious to you, but not your colleagues. Once at the hospital, quickly but carefully review the patient's labs,

L. Szczurek, DO, FACOS (✉)
Jefferson Health New Jersey, Cherry Hill, NJ, USA

H. Graves, MD
Vascular Surgery, Jefferson Health New Jersey, Voorhees, NJ, USA

© Springer International Publishing AG, part of Springer Nature 2018
K. Yoon-Flannery et al. (eds.), *A Surgeon's Path*,
https://doi.org/10.1007/978-3-319-78846-3_34

imaging, and history prior to speaking with the patient and family or calling in the operating room staff. You need to make sure all of the information given to you up until this point is accurate and that the patient does need an operation and what operation is going to be planned.

Next you will need to obtain informed consent, reviewing all of the risks and benefits of the planned surgery with the patient and the patient's family. Take time to make sure that you answer any questions that the patient and family have, and also review options other than surgery with them. You will quickly learn that not all surgical cases are black and white. If you think there is a high potential for morbidity and mortality, be honest and tell the patient and family. Make sure everyone is prepared for all the possibilities, including death. It is also prudent to establish a do not resuscitate (DNR) status prior going to the operating room. Most importantly, make sure you are carrying out the wishes of the patient. Do not force a surgery on someone that does not want to be operated on. If you think the patient will not survive the operation, you do not have to offer the procedure, however, be prepared to explain this to the patient and family.

Once you know what emergent operation that you will be performing, you will need to utilize your operating room's emergency add-on policy. During the day, you may need to call the head of anesthesia and the nurse running the OR board. During the night, your first callout of bed should be to the on-call OR nurse so she can call in anesthesia, the PACU nurse, the scrub nurse, the OR circulator, and support staff, including fluoroscopy or perfusion. You may be required to speak to other surgeons who also have simultaneous emergencies and work to prioritize who goes first.

You should also contact the anesthesia and operating room staff to make sure that they have all the equipment you need available. Think about all of the potential items required for the surgery (i.e., catheters, sutures, drains, staplers, hernia meshes, dressings, etc.), and make sure that the staff has all of the equipment in the OR room before you start so that the circulating nurse does not have to keep running out of the room to gather things. Not only will the constant disruption aggravate the staff but you as well when you have to keep waiting for the nurse to return with the items you need to continue the procedure.

The goal of the surgery is to fix the problem and get the patient off of the operating room table safely. Review the step of the procedure in your head before you start the case, and if needed, consult a book, video, or colleague for any last minute tips. If you are struggling during the case and need help, whether it is a quick question, an extra set of hands or a more senior surgeon's assistance, DO NOT BE AFRAID or TOO PROUD to call. Every surgeon has had this experience at some time in their career. Remember, you should always choose what is safe for the patient. You will never be faulted for doing a safe operation or calling for help.

Lastly, take each emergent case as a learning opportunity. Think about what you did right and what you could have done differently. Once you have evaluated the case for yourself, it can be helpful to discuss the case with a colleague. It can be useful to get another perspective; however, remember that everyone was trained differently and there is not just one way to solve a problem. That being said, gain as much as you can from each experience, because your career is going to be full of emergencies!

Chapter 35
How to Avoid Disasters in the Operating Room

Introduction

Of all the apprehensions of a new surgical attending, the most significant perceived fear by new grads is a scenario in which the circumstances of the procedure fall out of their control, with unintended consequences. Chief residents are some of the most confident surgeons in the OR because they have a great deal of experience but are still supervised by a teaching surgeon, i.e., they always have someone to back them up if the case becomes too difficult or if unexpected findings are encountered. I have been training residents for over 12 years and have been a program director for the majority of that time. My job is not only to keep residents out of trouble but also to teach them how to avoid trouble when their careers have moved beyond training.

This chapter is a simple, yet focused attempt to outline the barriers to safe, controlled surgery, with an emphasis on the challenges of new grads. Most residents enter the job market these days after additional fellowship training and are lucky enough to have partners to assist them as necessary. Some, however, do pursue general surgery in rural areas without fellowship training and without significant mentorship. Regardless of your circumstance, the safety of your patients should be your number one focus when starting your first job. Avoiding trouble in the OR is critical in maintaining patient well-being. I've outlined my steps to maintain a consistent, safe environment for my patients. They include:

Step 1. Practice preparedness
Step 2. Optimize team dynamics
Step 3. Focus on aftercare

L. Balsama, DO, FACS
General Surgery Residency Program, General and Bariatric Surgery,
Rowan University School of Osteopathic Medicine, Stratford, NJ, USA
e-mail: balsamlo@rowan.edu

© Springer International Publishing AG, part of Springer Nature 2018
K. Yoon-Flannery et al. (eds.), *A Surgeon's Path*,
https://doi.org/10.1007/978-3-319-78846-3_35

Step 1. Practice Preparedness

Preparedness is perhaps the most important component for a successful and safe surgery. Hospital culture has changed greatly over the past decade. We are now asked to see patients within 30 days of an operation and also perform a complete history and physical on the patient prior to entering the operating room, whereas these rules were not always in place historically. They are meant to protect the patient from being the victim of a mistake, but they can only be useful if the surgeon not only follows the letter of the law but also the spirit of the law. The surgeon must foster a culture that places patient safety and concern above surgeon pride or authority. The OR team must be able to approach a surgeon with concerns if there are discrepancies in the patient's information or findings.

Proper preparedness, from a surgeon's point of view, starts with a **pre-op note**. This moment of reflection allows the surgeon to carefully review the patient's information in a logical, progressive manner, which I recommend should be done in a narrative form. I have personally changed my intended procedure more than once, after reviewing the facts of a patient's case. A pre-op note should include the chief complaint, an abbreviated summary of pertinent findings, and what the intended surgery may include. It should also document discussions had by the patient, the patient's family, and the surgeon, prior to consent. The consent should duplicate the intended procedure on the preoperative note. This seemingly short, discrete documentation may seem redundant, but it is essential to staying out of troubling situations. It provides *your* expectations of the surgery, as opposed to the consent, which gives the *patient's* expectations of it, meaning that a preoperative note should be more explanatory and precise than a simple explanation of the procedure.

Here is an example of how I have seen a junior resident write a pre-op note:

Pre-op Dx: Cholecystitis in a 43 y/o female
Consent signed
Antibiotics on hold for the O.R.
Normal labs

So, certainly, this very straightforward patient may not require a long pre-op note. But if my resident is just writing down what they feel they already know, they are just skimming the surface of the note. I try to guide my residents to look deeper, to ask themselves about decision-making processes that are made with each patient to ensure that the correct procedure is done safely. Does this patient need a cholangiogram? Or a preoperative cardiac workup? Are there any unexpected findings on the ultrasound? Any variance in the answers to these questions creates new therapeutic avenues.

Here is how I want my residents to write a pre-op note:

This patient is a 43 y/o female with no previous medical or surgical issues presenting with right upper quadrant pain yesterday, first episode. Findings include abdominal tenderness in RUQ, WBC 11, total bilirubin 0.7, normal EKG and ultrasound findings of gallstones with slight gallbladder wall thickening, and a liver cyst. Intended procedure is a laparoscopic cholecystectomy, possible open cholecystectomy, and possible cholangiogram. Risks and complications of the procedure explained in depth to the patient and her husband. She and her husband are agreeable to proceed. Pre-op antibiotics to be given within 1 h of procedure.

In this above example, it is obvious to me that the surgeon looked at the pertinent findings and reviewed the necessary results to think of every possibility in this case, even though it is a simple one.

In keeping with an accurate preoperative assessment, a history and physical should be done prior to any procedure. There are obvious advantages to this requirement. I have seen patients that omitted recent falls or traumas prior to a bariatric procedure. Obviously, if they cannot walk, their risk of developing a DVT or PE increases dramatically. In fact, they may have already developed a DVT by being immobile since the accident. Another common finding may be the development of an arrhythmia, such as atrial fibrillation, prior to surgery that must be first addressed. Questions that I use commonly when interviewing my patients include: "Have there been any changes in your health since the last time we met?" "Any recent traumas or accidents?" "Any recent illnesses?" I have found that patients do not consider falls or traumas to be a medical condition. Some patients are surprised when I ask these questions, especially if I just saw a patient recently. A lot can happen in a week!

Re-acquaint yourself with the region of the body that will be addressed. On physical exam, note any scars or changes in the findings of the pathology. If a hernia is no longer palpable, make sure that your original findings were accurate. Don't be hesitant to ask the patient to stand up, or change positions, to confirm that the pathology is still present. I do mark hernias, even when it is not required, because it helps me choose my incision site. This marking may be slightly different when the patient is in different positions. Also, because there may be a delay between seeing a patient in the office and operating on them, make sure that you are still able to palpate a mass, if present, as lymph nodes notoriously may disappear if they are simply reactive. Make sure that the patient is still able to detect the finding, such as a mass or lymph node, prior to proceeding. Sometimes you may also discover new findings that could delay the intended procedure, such as rash or infection. Obviously, if a patient has a new cast or splint, this must be explained by the patient and noted on the chart. For elective cases, this finding may result in a postponement.

It is always a good habit to quickly review a procedure prior to the case, even as a seasoned surgeon. This is especially helpful with unusual or rare cases that still fall into the scope of a surgeon's practice. An example might be a Heller myotomy, a gastric cancer resection, or a femoral hernia repair by a general surgeon. I always find it surprising when my medical students answer questions wrong in the OR, not because I think that they are easy questions but because there is such an extensive access to information in our modern era. Social media contains scientific literature, diagrams, and videos on all operative procedures, with many different techniques and excellent descriptions of anatomy. In a matter of minutes, a medical student may watch four different videos describing techniques for a particular surgery, all with full explanations…on their phone! I would also highly recommend the same videos for practicing surgeons. It keeps your mind open to improve your technique and provide alternatives to the techniques you learned as a resident. The best surgeons review anatomy constantly and are open to newer, better techniques.

Another way to prepare properly for an operation is to consider any specialists that may have a role in the procedure. Examples may include urologists to place stents prior to an elective colon procedure or gynecologists that may be involved in evaluating pelvic cysts or masses seen on CT. Always contact your specialty colleagues as soon as you know that you are doing the case, as it is respectful to their time commitment. If you think that a particular procedure may require help from another specialist, try to schedule the case (if possible) for a weekday when that particular specialist is also operating. It is often difficult, especially in a small hospital, to find a gynecologist or urologist at a moment's notice. Delaying the intraoperative consult as you wait for the specialist to arrive will result in your patient enduring additional time under anesthesia, which has obvious drawbacks. Also, learn to broaden your techniques so that you may avoid the need for specialist involvement, when possible. A good example may be to familiarize yourself with intraoperative cholangiograms to rule out common duct stones, thereby negating the need for GI consultation in borderline cases.

Anticipate what materials you may need for a case, especially when first starting in a new hospital. You may be very shocked to find out that a particular instrument that you used very regularly in training is not available at your new hospital of practice! It is always a good idea to take material lists from your hospital of training so that you may give a copy of them to the nursing supervisor in your new hospital. It provokes great anxiety in surgeons when they are forced to use unfamiliar instrumentation or, worse, have no suitable substitutes for a particular instrument or material. Most hospitals, I find, are very accommodating to your needs when you are first starting, but be open to substitute materials and learn the limitations of your available resources, just in case.

Step 2. Optimize Team Dynamics

The first thing that I learned when I started as an attending surgeon (at a different hospital from where I had previously trained) was that resources might vary, not only in materials but also in personnel. Just as we all know that different surgeons bring different talents into the OR, so do your OR personnel. Any given scrub tech, anesthesiologist, nurse anesthetist, or circulating nurse may be new or experienced, strict or relaxed, engaged or lackadaisical. The biggest hurdle when starting in a new hospital is to figure out the strengths and weaknesses of your OR team on any given day. It is always a good idea to recognize that you are part of a "team" and that you should familiarize yourself with that team and be very communicative during the case to avoid problems. Introduce yourself to any personnel whom you are not familiar. This not only promotes good chemistry in the OR, but it also puts forth a level of approachability. Even though you may find it hard to believe that your coworkers may be afraid of you or intimidated by you, sometimes it is, very much, the case. Your staff will be more likely to express concerns to you if they find you to be friendly and communicative.

Teach your team. This is important especially in close-knit community hospitals. Your staff will respect you and treat you well if you teach them *Before* the case what you might be doing and why. Again, those nurses, techs, and anesthesiologists that are working around you are curious and want to know about the patient's condition and what you might be doing for them. They also will appreciate if you tell them beforehand what steps you will take and what instruments you might use. It does not shed good light on your demeanor, as a surgeon, if you become angry or frustrated when certain resources are not available or that when staff is not familiar with your technique. Exercise some empathy for your coworkers, and verbalize your own style and technique so that your staff is ready and willing to help you.

When things go wrong in the OR, the mood and actions of those around you may be compromised based on your own mood and actions. Stress is amplified in the OR if the surgeon is visibly shaken. I have met many surgeons that practice varying types of relaxation techniques to avoid confrontation with other coworkers or embarrassing moments of losing one's patience in the OR. If you want your colleagues to continue to be confident in your abilities as a surgeon, it is important that you "keep your cool" in all circumstances. It is OK to show some emotion and urgency. It is NOT OK to place blame, patronize, belittle, or chastise a coworker in the heat of the moment. It is not productive and will only breed contempt and disrespect. That said, we all have instigated, witnessed, or been subject to such indiscretions. Be mindful of your mood and constantly monitor your affect toward others. The most respected surgeons are those that remain professional and controlled, even in tough situations.

You will, no doubt, have your favorite personnel and your not-so-favorite personnel in the OR. As a professional surgeon, you do not get to choose (most of the time) who will be in your OR for a particular day. It is important to remain neutral to staff, if possible, and not show favoritism. This is sometimes harder than you might think to accomplish. A staff member will be much more accommodating to you if they feel that they are being treated fairly, in relation to their peers.

Step 3. Focus on Aftercare

As all residents and practicing surgeons realize, aftercare is very important in ensuring that your intervention is lasting and beneficial. Implementation of aftercare begins in the operating room. Your preoperative thoughts and preparations may be thorough and complete for the operation itself, but there are additional considerations for the patient when completing the procedure to ensure the patient has a smooth transition to their next destination, may it be recovery room, home, or ICU. Staying out of trouble sometimes involves the interventions that you initiate at the end of surgery or in your postoperative orders. Unfortunately, I've seen many a good operation fail due to lack of attention to detail in the recovery room, on the floor, or in the unit. It is extremely important to continue to think of ways of optimizing your patient's outcome, even though the operative portion of their therapy is drawing to a close.

When your operation is concluding and you are beginning to close your incisions, you should be going through a "postoperative checklist" in your mind. This should include a number of variables, and they are case specific. A few examples may be:

"Have I checked for sponges?" (In most cases of retained sponges, the sponge count is "correct" by staff.)

"Have I rechecked any areas of nuisance bleeding to ensure that they are controlled?" (There is nothing so frustrating as taking a patient back for active bleeding.)

"Does my patient require a binder?" (Not just hernias, any large abdominal incision will make the patient more comfortable; they will require less pain medicine and be less likely to develop a hernia.)

"Is my patient waking up violently?" (Always good advice to apply pressure to a new hernia repair if patient is coughing excessively during anesthesia recovery.)

"Does my patient require a drain? And if so, what kind and how should it be handled by nursing?" (Think especially with perforated ulcer or bile leak, in which a drain is most effective and supported.)

"Will this ostomy retract? Or are there any techniques that may prevent this?" (Always make sure the colon can be withdrawn 3–4 cm PAST the skin edge before closing the abdomen, in an ostomy case.)

"Does this patient need retention sutures?" "Would this patient be better served with feeding access/G-tube?" (Both of these previous questions should be asked for a patient with poor nutritional status or on steroids.)

"Will this wound get infected? Should I use a VAC or open dressing, instead of closing skin?' (Think of this especially with dirty cases, such as colon perforation.)

"Have I instilled adequate amounts of local anesthesia to bridge the patient to recovery?" (The skin and peritoneum are the most densely innervated tissues of the abdomen/focus your injections in these two layers.)

"Have I verified the position of the drain/NGT, etc.?"

Be satisfied that you were not only thorough during the case but also thorough at the conclusion of the case, when the mood is light and focus on details may be less rigorous. I would say that, of all the facets of residency training, this aftercare part is the least taught but the most important in ensuring quality outcomes.

Certainly, although you will be diligent in your postoperative care, there are patients that will still need reoperation due to complications. In these circumstances, surgeons need to recognize that their own bias of "surgeon pride" may delay necessary intervention. Most surgeons don't want to acknowledge that a patient is having a complication, sometimes even though it may be plainly obvious. I've seen this many times, with many colleagues. I have succumbed to this myself in certain circumstances. The real problem with this situation is that most complications are better treated early, not late. For example, after a patient undergoes a sigmoid resection with primary anastomosis, they may complain of increasing pain and lack of bowel function. CT demonstrates a "collection with contrast" adjacent to the anastomosis. Many surgeons may try to handle that problem "conservatively" with percutaneous drainage, but a breakdown or nonhealing of a fresh anastomosis usually is best treated with urgent surgical intervention. That problem is not going away! In these circumstances, the best advice is to swallow your pride, talk to your colleagues, and go over your options with the patient. Always include the patient in your discussions. It is well known that patients are less likely to bring lawsuits forth if they are well informed, even in the face of unexpected complications. They will also continue to trust you and respect your decisions if they feel that you are being open and honest.

In conclusion, I hope that you find this chapter useful, not only by reading it once but reviewing it from time to time so that you may reflect on the parts of your practice that may become overly "routine." Understand that you will mature as a surgeon and improve your abilities to anticipate problems, but the disadvantage of this is that we still may be lacking in thoroughness in some situations. This is because we have the experience of those situations in the past and expect the same results. Don't do this! The beauty and art of surgery is that our patients continually present challenges to us that are new and unique, no matter what our experience tells us. Excellent surgeons realize that no case is routine, they focus on the nuances of the case in order to learn something new and improve their care of patients. If, instead, we focus only on the superficial information and generalities of cases, we are sure to get into troubling situations. Stay focused, stay thorough, and enjoy the art of surgery.

Chapter 36
When to Ask for Help

Linda Szczurek

The answer to the question of when to ask for help is probably the easiest of all the topics in this book. If the thought of asking for help pops into you head for any reason whatsoever, you should rely on your instinct and ask!

You should never be afraid or too proud to ask for help. You are still very young in your career and in a totally new environment. Everyone from the Chief of Surgery at the hospital to the parking lot attendant was new at some point. Most of the other physicians and staff at the hospital will be more than willing to help with anything from directions to needing extra assistance during a case. As interns, I'm certain that we all got a page on our first night of call for some problem that we weren't sure about. We quickly learned that there are many resources other than Google from which you can find the answer. The easiest way is usually to ask someone else who has more experience than you. This could be the resident on call or many times the nurse who is taking care of the patient who has also been doing her job since before you could walk.

For most surgeons it takes about 4–5 years as an attending before you are comfortable with most cases. Of course, this varies depending on many factors including your personal skill level, the number of cases of that type you did during training and are currently performing, and the breath of cases that you choose to perform. In my practice, I perform most bread and butter general surgery cases such as cholecystectomies, hernia repairs, and colon surgeries. There are certain procedures that over the past few years I stopped doing because I was busy with others. In this case, I will refer the patient to see one of my partners who is better qualified to take care of the problem. I never want to be caught in a situation where I perform a surgery that I have little experience with or do not feel comfortable with and the patient has a complication. It will not look very good if there is a lawsuit and you have to explain why you chose to operate on the patient even though you have only done

L. Szczurek, DO, FACOS
Jefferson Health New Jersey, Cherry Hill, NJ, USA
e-mail: linda.szczurek@jefferson.edu

© Springer International Publishing AG, part of Springer Nature 2018
K. Yoon-Flannery et al. (eds.), *A Surgeon's Path*,
https://doi.org/10.1007/978-3-319-78846-3_36

this procedure once in the past year instead of referring the patient to your partner or another surgeon nearby who performs the surgery on a regular basis. Remember, your primary goal is patient safety.

For elective surgeries, planning ahead and asking for help is much easier. You will have a complete history and physical examination for the patient and radiology/lab studies if needed. This information can be very helpful prior to surgery. Since you have more time with elective office patients, you can consult other sources such as textbooks, journal articles, or videos. If you think the surgery will be very complex because the patient has had multiple surgeries in the past, the anatomy looks difficult on imaging studies, or the case is not something you have had a lot of experience doing, you can easily speak with one of your more senior partners about the case and ask your office to schedule the case for both of you. This will help avoid a potential disaster in the future if you really do need help. If you are currently looking for your first job as an attending, I recommend asking your future potential colleagues about their view on this topic. Will they be willing to double scrub cases with you or come in at night when you are on call to help if you are having a problem or not? It is very stressful to start a new job but to do this knowing that you have no back up if needed could make the situation much worse.

Surgery is not black and white, and patients always present differently. Some will have the classic textbook presentation and others will be much more complicated. I work with five other surgeons in my group. My senior partner has been practicing for almost 30 years, and I am the newest, 7 years, and whenever there is a difficult case, we run it past one another to get another opinion. It helps to build confidence when you first start to get confirmation from a more experienced surgeon that your plan for a patient is appropriate and that you have back up if needed. There are many other sources that you can go to for advice in the planning process including reviewing the images with the radiologist directly or calling a friend or mentor from residency or fellowship that you trust and to get their opinion.

In general, if you feel like you are in over your head, feel you have a complication/mistake, or feel you need more insight or expertise, you SHOULD call for help. This applies to both the operating room and office. Asking for assistance is not a sign of weakness or lack of knowledge. Your colleagues and staff will respect you more for not being afraid to ask for help rather than watching you struggle too proud or arrogant making an unsafe decision leading to patient harm. Being too proud or arrogant will never end well for yourself or your patient.

Chapter 37
Finding the Balance of Letting Residents Operate While Managing Patient Safety

Linda Szczurek

There are many benefits of accepting a new job at a teaching hospital. Residents can be very helpful with patient care and providing assistance in the operating room. However, if you are reading this book, you are probably still in residency/fellowship or just finishing and you remember exactly what it was like to do all of these tasks hoping that you will get your reward in the OR by "getting to do the case." Gone are the days when the attending surgeon allows the resident to operate on a patient while he/she sits in the lounge drinking a cup of coffee. Medicare laws require surgeons to be present and scrubbed for the majority of the surgery and many hospital bylaws contain similar mandates.

Finding a balance between letting residents operate while maintaining patient safety will be likely be one of your greatest challenges not only when you first start as an attending but throughout your career at a teaching institution. This is because both you and each of the residents are continually evolving. Over the years with more experience, you will be more confident in your skills allowing residents to play a more active role in the OR. The residents will all be very different in skill level, knowledge, and progression. Not to mention that residents are frequently changing rotations/services operating with different attending surgeons, and it can be hard to keep track of an individual residents' abilities.

Think back to all of the attending surgeons that you worked with during your training. I'm sure there were great differences in the level of freedom surgeons let you have in the OR. You will need to figure out where on this spectrum you will likely fall, and this may change over time. Some of the adjustments to your new role as an attending will also affect the residents. They will need to understand that you are "NEW" and still learning just as they are. You may actually need to explain this to the residents so that they understand your situation. You need to learn to operate on your own first before you can be an effective teaching attending. I do not

L. Szczurek, DO, FACOS
Jefferson Health New Jersey, Cherry Hill, NJ, USA
e-mail: linda.szczurek@jefferson.edu

© Springer International Publishing AG, part of Springer Nature 2018
K. Yoon-Flannery et al. (eds.), *A Surgeon's Path*,
https://doi.org/10.1007/978-3-319-78846-3_37

recommend turning cases over to residents until you are completely comfortable doing them yourself.

This may mean that in the beginning, the more senior residents will shy away from scrubbing with you because they may not get to participate very much during the surgery. However, they will soon be in your shoes and realize why this is the case. Fortunately, this can prove beneficial to both you and the junior residents. Teaching the basic skills and steps in a procedure to a junior residents is an excellent way for the junior resident to learn as well as for you to become more confident in your own skills.

As you become more comfortable in your attending role and are ready to start allowing residents to play a more active role in the operating room, the next step will be learning to assess a resident's ability. This can be very difficult because each resident will very different; one PGY-3 resident may function at a level of a PGY-4 as far as knowledge and skills but another PGY-3 in the same program may only function at the level of a PGY-2 resident. It is important for you to be familiar with the level for each resident so that you can determine how much and which cases you can allow a resident to perform while ensuring patient safety.

How do you accomplish this? Good news is that surgery residency is 5–7 years long, giving you ample time to get to know the residents that you work with. One of the easiest ways to help you figure out a resident's level other than direct observation of their OR skills is to start by asking the resident questions. Do they know what case they are doing? Do they know the patient's history? Did they look at imaging studies if applicable? What are the steps of the planned surgery? What is the anatomy? What equipment do you need? What are the potential risks or complications of the procedure and what can be done to avoid or fix them? If the resident does not know the answers to these questions, he/she is either unprepared or the case is above his/her level and he/she should not be participating in any of the significant steps of the surgery for patient safety reasons. The patient and their safety is ultimately your responsibility so it is also your responsibility to judge residents' abilities and amount of participation.

There are many other factors that play into the amount of resident participation other than resident level that you may have never thought about: the type of surgery, you would not let a first year resident do the same amount of a major surgery such as a laparoscopic colon resection as you would the chief resident; comorbidities and body habitus of a patient, it is much easier to operate on a thin patient than a patient that is morbidly obese; schedule, allowing resident participation and teaching take extra operating time (sometimes you may have to explain to a resident that is has nothing to do with his or her skill level but you are already running late and his or her role in the case will be limited); time of day, resident participation is often limited during emergency cases that occur in the middle of the night (everyone in the room is tired including you, the resident, the OR staff, and the anesthetist, and no one wants to stand and watch as you try to teach or let a resident struggle through a portion of the surgery at 2 AM); and patient request, most patients are very happy to have a resident involved in their care, but attending surgeons do get requests from patients on a regular basis that the resident is allowed in the OR room to watch or hold retractors but the patient does not want them do any of the operation. In this situation, you should abide by the patient's wishes and explain the reason to the resident.

The attending/resident relationships function best with mutual trust and respect and with each individual realizing their own limitations and tolerances. As a teaching attending, you must be confident that you can fix any problem that a resident may cause. If you cannot do this, you should not be allowing the resident to be doing this portion of the surgery. In reverse, the residents must trust that you are teaching them proper patient care and techniques and that you will be able to fix something should they have a misstep during the procedure.

When you notice that a resident is struggling in the operating room, taking over a case can actually turn into an excellent teaching opportunity. You can explain or teach a resident a new technique so that the next time, he/she will be more prepared and know what or how to do.

Although choosing to work in a teaching hospital comes with a responsibility of educating residents, medical students, and fellows, your ultimate goal is always patient safety. Fortunately, over time and as you gain more experience, finding a balance between resident participation in the OR and patient safety does get easier. It is not a process that will happen overnight, and it will not be a stress-free process. I can tell you from experience that helping to educate the next generation of surgeons is well worth the risk.

Chapter 38
Choosing the Right Staff

Robert Neff and Marc Neff

In our experience the right staff is one of the most critical things that impacts a business and the overall success of the business. Staff members are on the front lines representing all of the professionals in the organization. It is likely that a patient's first interaction with an organization is through someone other than the provider, whether it is with the security guard in the front lobby, the receptionist, or the information technology (IT) department because they are having trouble making an online appointment. All of these interactions will inform the overall patient experience and impact the decision of the patient to come back.

The best way to find staff is through networking and personal connectoins. It seems odd in today's world where almost everything is done online that picking employees is best done through word of mouth. The biggest reason this is the case is because it quickly speeds up the screening process. If someone is recommended to you via someone else, the person making the referral is essentially vouching for the good work of that employee. That immediately allows you to rule out some common concerns, which are hard to screen for, such as work ethic, past professional problems, etc.

Whether you find someone via a referral or other means, you will likely post the job on a website for people to apply. The first time we did this, it was shocking to see the types of resumes that were received. We have seen cases where office administrative assistants have applied to be physician leaders in a cardiology

R. Neff, BSc (✉)
Digital Innovation and Consumer Experience Group (DICE),
Thomas Jefferson University and Jefferson Health,
Philadelphia, PA, USA
e-mail: robert.neff@jefferson.edu

M. Neff, MD, FACS, FASMBS
Center for Surgical Weight Loss,
Jefferson Health New Jersey,
Cherry Hill, NJ, USA
e-mail: marc.neff@jefferson.edu

© Springer International Publishing AG, part of Springer Nature 2018
K. Yoon-Flannery et al. (eds.), *A Surgeon's Path*,
https://doi.org/10.1007/978-3-319-78846-3_38

department. When you look at the ease of applying to jobs online, you can see that candidates are rewarded for applying to as many jobs as they can. Even if they are not a fit for the job, they have the recruiter's attention and might be a fit for something else. Since there is no cost for them to apply, they have nothing lost but time—and if they are already unemployed, their time is not that valuable at that moment.

If you cannot find a staff member through an online website or word of mouth, there are always recruiting firms. These firms are hit-or-miss in our experience. The best ones specialize in finding people with a very specific skill set. These firms will often do much of the pre-vetting and screening, so that saves you some time sifting through possibly hundreds of resumes. These firms do cost quite a bit however, as typical fees are anywhere from 15% to 25% of the candidate's yearly salary as a finder's fee.

Once you have a candidate that may be a potential fit, you will want to interview that person. It is necessary during the interview to determine if the candidate has the skill set required for the job, but the best interviews go beyond simply determining basic qualifications. Additionally, you want to look for work ethic, values, ethics, and the personality of the candidate. Ensuring that the staff member has similar values and will uphold the mission of the organization is important. Further, ensuring that the existing team members and staff will work well together with the new hire is valuable. We often include the other staff in the interview process. It is good skill building for them but also allows them to feel a part of the process. Ultimately they will need to work with this person as well, and ensuring that they will have a rapport is important.

We often lament that when interviewing someone for a job, there may be one or two interviews, each an hour or so in length. During these few hours, you are expected to choose a person who you may spend the majority of your days with (often >8 h/day) and has a large impact on your overall professional success. In contrast, people spend years courting a spouse to make sure they have found the right person. The lesson here is to take your time and make the right hiring decisions. The wrong person cannot only underperform in his or her job but has the potential to negatively affect the rest of the staff and environment. It is better to keep a position open and have nobody than hire the wrong person.

When it comes to negotiating salary, we tend to prefer when candidates try to negotiate. It shows us they are not afraid to push the limits and that they believe in their own value. In general, we prefer paying people what they believe they are worth. If someone is requesting a salary that is out of our budget, but in line with market rates, we do not suggest trying to get them to work for less. That approach will leave you with an employee who will be less engaged and keeping their eyes focused on the next better opportunity.

Once the candidate has accepted the position, it is important to do your due diligence on him or her. This is where standard processes in an HR department can make the work easier, but if you are doing this yourself, you may want to consider looking at references, drug tests, and background screening and also having a probation period where the employment can be ended for any reason in the first 90 days.

Part Time, Temporary, or Contract Staff

In some cases, due to circumstances, it might be necessary to use contract or temporary staff. These staff members can often be provided through the same firms that provide recruitment services. These types of staff members are best to use in cases where you need a very specific skill set and you will only need it for a short period of time—such as doing a complex technical system upgrade. They might also be good for a more general skill set, but you need increased capacity (like more people to answer the phone) leading up to a big event.

If contract resources are used, you will want to consider a lot of the same type of issues you have while selecting regular staff, but you can know that it is easy to cancel these contract resources at the first sign of any issue—so there is a smaller risk to impacting the rest of your staff with a bad employee that is hard to get rid of.

If the contract resources you bring in will be there for a longer term, I would try—as much as possible—to not differentiate them from the rest of the staff in any significant way. You don't want to create a culture where there are two casts of employees. This will only add unnecessary challenges into the environment and hurt the culture.

Making Sure You Are Using Resources Effectively

Staff members require training, performance evaluation, paychecks, and direction. In some ways, your staff will be your family away from home, and you need to put them in the right environment to succeed. As Einstein said, "Everyone is a genius. But if you judge a fish by its ability to climb a tree, it will live its whole life believing that it is stupid." Applying this to your office means recognize the training and talent of your staff and giving them appropriate tasks.

Example: You have multiple unfilled needs in your office. You need a data collector, a person to review labs and answer patients postoperative questions, and a part-time scheduler. We always want more staff, but staff are expensive and you can't always have what you want. You review your resources. You have a medical assistant that is very good at her job and a nurse who is able to do just about anything. Fatal flaw here would be to give the medical assistant all the labs to review. That is not in her scope of practice. Maybe you could give her certain ones, with training, but you can't expect her to interpret labs as a trained physician would. You could delegate these to your nurse, but she's a very valuable employee, and her time may be better spent answering patients' questions than filling in wherever you need help.

Take the time to write down your needs. Discuss them with the other physicians in your office. Review them with your office manager. They may have suggestions and be able to help you assign the right resource for the right job. The goal is to work smarter, not harder. Don't get frustrated with your staff. That isn't going to help them be any more efficient.

Salaries

If you are an employed physician, much of the salary discussion related to your employees is out of your control. The fair market value of someone's position and training is the most important component. The years of training or loyalty to you isn't. For example, you sell your practice to your hospital and medical assistant is planning to come with you, but there's an issue, the salary. Even though they've worked for you for the past 10 years and received a bonus each and every year for exemplary performance, their level of training determines their compensation, and they will get paid the same as the medical assistant who has been employed for 1 or 2 years. It may not be fair, but that's the way it is.

If you are a private practice surgeon, then you need to know what the 25%, 50%, and 75% payments are for a person in that position, based on their degrees, years of training, and your geographic location. You may want to keep the reimbursement low at first, with appropriately timed reviews and increases in their pay, or maybe through yearly bonuses, but keep in mind that your office staff contributes to your overhead. If you reward loyalty and offer raises and bonuses excessively each and every year, pretty soon, you are going to have some pretty expensive staff that have outpriced themselves from the marketplace. Yes, you get what you pay for, but if your overhead starts to cost too much, your practice is going to implode.

We are personally fond of the idea of a bonus. It gives your employees an incentive for going to extra mile. In our previous lives as private practitioners, we were able to reward staff for going above and beyond. I think that encourages hard work. We would like to think that our staff is working as hard and as efficient as they can each and every day, but having a bonus structure would have made that question different.

Last point, you can't tell your staff not to talk about their salaries. You can't tell them that it causes conflict or that people can be fired for doing it. Under the National Labor Relations Act of 1935, all workers have the right to discuss their wages, hours, and other conditions of employment. Yes, it is true and your staff should certainly get to talk together about things that matter to them at work.

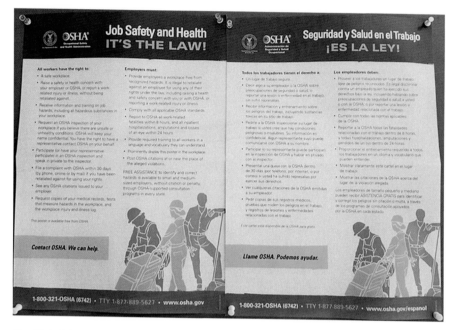

Fig. 38.1 Job safety and health posting

Important Employment Laws

We have addressed some of the laws that need to be followed with regard to employees. There are others. Your human resources department will address these if you are an employed physician, but it's up to you and your office manager if you are private.

Many states have posting requirements. For starters, you are going to need a workplace safety poster. Prepared by the Department of Labor, it informs employees of the protections of the Occupational Safety and Health Act. Then, you need a poster regarding the Fair Labor Standards Act, information about minimum wage, the Conscientious Employee Protection Act, family leave, information about harassment, and child labor laws. You also need information in other languages (Spanish). A picture of what is prominently displayed in our office kitchen is provided (Fig. 38.1).

Training Your Staff

An important part of running a successful surgical practice, whether you are employed or private, is training the right staff. You can't just find the right people for the job and turn them loose. Chaos will ensue. They need direction from you. A surefire way to disaster is to allow your staff to determine your practice of medicine.

Example: Mary is the your new medical assistant. She is well trained and interviewed well. You want her to help in your breast clinic. She has little familiarity with breast surgery. Take the time to sit down with her. It may sound trivial to you, but it is as vital as reviewing your own mammograms. Tell her what you want for new patients. For follow-ups. For in-office procedures. Don't assume she knows how to handle specimens. Don't assume that your current staff will train her. Script it. Tell her that you will review her interactions with you and the patients at the end of the first week. Give her the time from your schedule she needs to ask you questions and get appropriate feedback. Make these meetings frequent in the beginning, less frequent as time goes by and she is demonstrating appropriate growth. Your staff is an extension of you. Give them the time and attention they deserve, and let them be an extension of your talent.

Culture

An office culture is quite important, and one cannot underestimate how important it is to the employees. When you consider, again, that the staff might spend more of their life in the office than at home—you can begin to understand how seemingly little things can begin to matter quite a bit. There is always much in the news in the way of workplace culture and how to keep employees engaged. We tend to prefer to give as much control to the staff as we can to let them define the culture.

The culture includes everything from how people are treated, to what perks they get, to the physical space they occupy. Perks as simple as getting a new laptop, computer mouse, coffee mug, etc. can go a long way in keeping employees engaged. These things can certainly add up in cost depending on the size of an office—but if you consider the costs of recruiting new employees and staff turnover—spending a couple thousand extra dollars on this per year is small in comparison and it promotes a positive culture.

Within an organized group of people, subgroups will begin to form. People from similar backgrounds and with similar interests will tend to group and befriend each other. This is actually great, there is nothing better than getting to feel like you are with your friends all day at work. Early in our career, at one office we worked in, we became extremely friendly with two of our colleagues to the point we were sometimes referred to as the three amigos. That job was fantastic, as every day we looked forward to going to work to be with friends.

The most important about these groups or cliques that form is to be aware of them. You need to notice if they prevent people from getting work done or if some employees are excluded to the point they feel alone. This creates a bad environment and also a challenging place to get work done. In addition, to be aware of the cliques that form throughout your office, you should look at times and ways to get staff which don't always work together to know each other better. This can happen through special projects or team building activities. Cultivating a culture where it is painless for people to collaborate and communicate will go a long way to improving the overall success and efficiency of the office.

How to Evaluate Your Staff Performance

After you have chosen the right staff, trained them, and created the proper office environment, you have to determine how to evaluate their performance. For starters, determine, based on their job description and your needs, what will be the measures of their performance. For a physician's assistant, it may be the number of patients they have seen or their patient satisfaction scores. For a medical assistant, it could be less tangible such as how easy they make your office hours and if their entries into the electronic health record are correct. Set appropriate and transparent methods of assessing their progress and how often you will do it. These need to be private, one-on-one meetings, and the staff need to know your expectations ahead of time. The feedback should be constructive, positive, and with specific goals for the next assessment.

Example: Your secretary Toni has been working diligently for you for the past 2 months. She asks for an opportunity to review with her performance. It is reasonable and appropriate and you should have thought of this first. Regardless, you need to now plan out this meeting. Set up an outline. Focus on (1) measuring her performance, (2) giving her feedback, (3) giving her an opportunity for self-evaluation, (4) recognizing her strengths and areas for improvement, (5) setting up the next time for performance feedback, and (6) documenting her progress. The best evaluations will include goals for the employee and larger office goals that they contribute to. "I want my patients to feel like when they are speaking to you, they are the most important person in the world. If they think that, we will be the busiest practice around." It is ok to negotiate the goals and measurements together to get buy-in from your staff. And, again, documentation here, as with everything else, is important. A written evaluation provides clear evidence that your staff was involved and understood the requirements of their job and the measurements of their performance.

What to Do with Staff That Is Getting Burned Out

Burnout is a very common buzzword in healthcare today. It affects physicians and their staff alike. Patients' satisfaction is labeled paramount, but that has to be balanced with the patient you suspect is abusing narcotics. Patients want to be seen on time but that has to be balanced with completing the necessary information in the electronic health record. Patients want to not have their appointment delayed, but they sometimes forget that they needed a referral before they can even be seen in your office. And all of this was missed by your office staff.

The first part about burnout is to recognize it. Are your staff working appropriate hours? Are they getting a break for lunch? Is the volume of office work and phone calls reasonable and appropriate? Secondly, ask them. Make it private. Maybe they have something going on at home or outside of the office that is affecting their focus and concentration. Much of burnout is related to chronic stress, so you have to get at what are the stressors, be they exhaustion, lack of motivation, cynicism.

In terms of what to do about burnout for the physician, that is addressed elsewhere in this book, but two key points are to unplug and get organized. With regard to unplugging, it has to do with work seeping into family time, vacations, or basically non-work time. In other words, don't text your staff when they aren't at work unless it's a complete emergency. Let them focus on their non-work life. Second, with regard to organization, burned out staff start missing things, and their performance suffers. Help them to create lists and prioritize. Put systems in place to remind them what to do and when to do it.

Challenging Workplace Issues

Romance in the workplace is a like a flower-covered minefield. People spend a majority of their waking hours at work, so it is natural that the people you see daily, with whom you have a lot in common with, start to lead into some special chemistry. It can be exciting to date someone that knows the demands of your job and someone that you know well. It's even easier to meet someone at work you like, that you share many experiences with, than meeting some random person at a bar or party. There are, however, some very specific pitfalls. First off, the romance is unlikely to stay quiet and likely to become everybody's business in your office, the subject of much rumor and speculation. Second, the romance is likely to affect job performance. Longer lunches together or staff sneaking off to be alone. Lastly, the potential legal consequences, if one party wants to end the relationship but the other doesn't, and they are of differing positions of authority, a sexual harassment claim could be on the horizon.

Another challenging workplace issue is when fights develop between staff members. You are a surgeon, you aren't a kindergarten teacher, and you don't want to have to be an unpaid referee in a fight, right? Wrong. You have the responsibility to speak up if the work is not getting done and you notice why. First off, be careful how you get involved. It is ok to allow venting and empathy, but don't take sides, you don't know the full story. Second, don't get involved with gossip. That won't help with anything and likely only make matters worse. Your office is like your second family, and feeding rumors about what may or may not be happening won't help anyone. Thirdly, make it clear how the fighting is affecting the office efficiency. How it's distracting everyone from getting things done and, in the end, making more work for everyone. Lastly, know your limits. You aren't a trained mediator, that's what human resources department and office managers are for.

The last challenging workplace issue to address here is harassment. The Fair Employment Law governs harassment in the workplace. Harassment is illegal if it singles a person out because of race, color, creed, ancestry, national origin, age, disability, sex, marital status, sexual orientation, and arrest or conviction record. Harassment may include verbal abuse, offensive cartoons, materials, or rude jokes and is not a few isolated incidents but a pattern of degrading conduct. Sexual harassment involves unwelcome sexual advances, verbal and physical conduct of a sexual nature, when such conduct is made a condition of employment or when acceptance is used as the basis for decisions affecting an employee's job, like job advancement. Harassment occurs when there is a disparity of power, and there are plenty of disparities in a physician's office. As an employer, you are responsible for harassment between coworkers if you know about the conduct and fail to take immediate appropriate corrective action.

Poor Performance and Firing Staff

When an employee is not performing as expected, either having challenges completing their work or other problems which are preventing them from being effective in their role, the most important thing is to begin to document the issues for your own records. Next, it is preferred to have a discussion with the employee and draft a performance improvement plan (PIP) which outlines areas for improvement that are required and some actions which the employee can take to improve in those areas. If everything goes well, following the plan will allow the employee to improve and become a more efficient and valuable member of your staff. If things don't go well, we are into a darker territory.

There are a lot of terms that are used when someone leaves a company against their own will. Sometimes it is because the employee has done something wrong—but many other times business circumstances require the business to reduce the number of employees. My personal favorite term is "downsized," but other common terms are being fired, "let go," "laid off," or being part of a "reduction in force." Typically, being fired refers to cases where an employee is asked to leave a company because he or she has done something wrong or has not met expectations. In these cases, the firing is often the culmination of a process or plan where you have been working with the employees to improve their performance, but they have not been able to improve to your satisfaction. Due to this, in most instances when an employee is fired, it does not come a surprise to them.

No manager or superior ever wants to fire someone. It is challenging to lose an employee for the business and very impactful to that person. Many times there may be a temptation to keep an existing employee and hope that things get better. The best argument against this is the ramifications for your other employees. It is likely that they notice problems with their coworkers' performance and keeping that person on staff makes more work for them. It also sends the message that you tolerate poor performance and you may see your other staff picking up some of those same behaviors.

Chapter 39
How to Be Smart with Case Selection

Gustavo Lopes

The first year as a surgical attending is likely the most challenging year of your medical career. The transition from resident to surgical attending is a difficult one, and even more difficult today than the past. The decisions you make during this time will set the tone for the remainder of your career. The experience can launch a budding career or act as a drag on your practice for years to come.

During training, each resident is so busy learning each of their mentor's individual techniques that he or she spends very little time developing his or her own. When making decisions as a resident, one acts based on the methods of that patient's attending surgeon. This happens from suture selection in the operating room to managing drains and diets on the floor. As a resident, you may have memorized ten different varied and nuanced ways of managing a nasogastric tube. The day you graduate, those decisions are now yours like they were never fully before. It may surprise you the first time you hesitate when asked what suture you like for a particulate task. You'll remember what each of your attendings would pick. But what would "I" like to use? You will be faced with hundreds of decisions like this, big and small.

One of the most important decisions you will face is regarding case selection. You will do this in a general sense as well as an individual basis. How you do this will ultimately define what your practice is and does. It will also shape the perceptions about you as a surgeon and the work you do.

As a resident, the scope of your practice was the scope of your attendings' practice, your service, and your hospital. Whatever cases were on the board, you did. Now you must decide what type of cases you want to perform, and more importantly, do not want to perform, and shape your practice accordingly. Some of this will happen naturally by the decisions you have already made, such as whether or not to get fellowship training. Even so, you must decide how wide or narrow the

G. Lopes, DO
General, Laparoscopic, and Robotic Surgery, Chairman Department of Surgery,
Martin Health System, Stuart, FL, USA

© Springer International Publishing AG, part of Springer Nature 2018
K. Yoon-Flannery et al. (eds.), *A Surgeon's Path*,
https://doi.org/10.1007/978-3-319-78846-3_39

scope of your practice will be. There will be elements out of your control in this regard. The makeup of the market you decide to start your career will affect how your practice develops. If you are a general surgeon practicing in an area saturated with fellowship trained breast surgeons, for example, it may be an uphill battle to make that a significant part of your practice. The appeal for a patient to see, or physician to refer to a subspecialist is strong. But, with time and effort, it can be done. On the other hand, if there is a deficiency of subspecialist or interest in one area of surgery, that may be an opportunity to quickly establish yourself and fill that void.

Simply start with what you would like to do. Make a list of procedures you want to be doing. Now ask, will this be enough to sustain a practice. For most of us, the answer is probably not. Make a list of procedures you are qualified to perform and willing to do. Hopefully, this list is now long enough to generate plenty of surgery to keep you busy. It is better not to be too picky in the beginning while you are building a practice. Being available goes a long way to building good will with referring doctors and a reputation of being a "go to" surgeon. You can always narrow your focus over time as your practice grows.

Give the procedure list to your office staff. This is a helpful resource as they process new referrals. They can schedule patients you can treat and quickly defer the ones you can't. There is no need for you to see patients that need surgeries you don't perform and have diseases you don't treat. Your time is valuable and your office appointments are limited. You want to maximize the chances that your new patients will be surgical patients; you are a surgeon after all. Patients' time is also valuable, and it should not require visits with multiple specialists, when one would do. Revisit your list from time to time and adjust if needed.

Once you have decided how your practice will look like in a general sense, you will be faced with decisions regarding individual case selection. These decisions are often much more difficult. There are a number of factors to consider as you decide whether you want to operate on a patient, some of which are patient-centric, while others will be procedure-centric.

Within the scope of your specialty and practice, there may be specific procedures you choose to avoid. You must carefully consider the resources available to you and determine if they are adequate to perform certain cases. If you are in a small community hospital without robust interventional radiology and critical care support, performing a Whipple procedure may not be the smartest idea, even if you are perfectly capable of performing the surgery. Additionally, you will need partners willing and able to back you up. If your partners don't perform the procedure and are not qualified to manage some of your patients, you will be essentially on call 24/7 for those patients. If these are fixable problems, then you hold off on doing those procedures until you have placed appropriate measures to handle them. If this cannot be done, you are better off transferring those cases to an institution that can handle them. Remember, it's not just the racecar driver but the entire pit crew and team that run the race. It may be very difficult to give up those cases, but performing them without appropriate support will be even more difficult.

Individual patients will present their own unique challenges. If it's an emergency call case, you may not have much choice in the matter. However, elective cases are different and difficult cases should be considered carefully. You don't have to take on the giant incisional hernia with loss of domain in a status post heart transplant patient your first year out. Maybe you never do. It is acceptable and smart to defer extremely difficult cases to a more experienced surgeon as you start off. It is worse for the patients and your career to collect a group of disaster cases you weren't quite ready for. This isn't to say that cherry-picking and dumping problem cases to others is the goal. As time goes on, you will have the confidence and experience to tackle the most difficult surgical problems. But to think you will be at that point on day one is unrealistic. If you are lucky enough to have a trusted and experienced partner available, ask for help. You can keep the case and learn from them, best of both worlds.

When deciding the approach you should take for a surgery, keep all options available. In the age of minimally invasive surgery for just about everything, it is easy to forget the tried and true open approach. Sometimes trying to do too much laparoscopically or sticking with it too long can create more problems which can easily snowball. If the case calls for converting to open, convert early. If the case calls for doing it open from the start, do it open. Don't be a hero, be a good general surgeon. Maximize your chance of having a good result and don't apologize for it. This is especially true in the beginning of your career, but don't forget it later in your career.

Remember, the impression you make in the first few months of a job will stick with you for years. Make decisions with the patient in mind and know yourself as a surgeon. Be realistic. Be safe. Be smart. Do that and you will grow as a surgeon and your practice will grow with you.

Chapter 40
Building Your Practice

John D. Paletta

Introduction

The task of turning your medical practice into a successful business venture can be overwhelming. Now that you are going about the business of setting up your new medical practice, you have to reach out to the referring doctors in town and somehow get the word out to potential patients that there is an excellent new surgeon in town—you!

Rest assured, there are many ways to build your practice and plenty of people who are willing to give you advice in this area. Learning what it takes to build a successful practice is a little bit like surgical training. You will be exposed to many different ideas, techniques, and tips—some you will adopt, and others you will discard as you become more comfortable with the process.

This chapter will introduce some ideas that may be useful for practice introduction and development. You may not feel comfortable with all of these techniques, and that is perfectly fine! Pick out the ones that make sense to you, use them, or modify them as you see fit. Some of these ideas will mesh perfectly with your personality, and they will help you to introduce yourself to the medical community in your new town and to productively utilize your free time early in the life of your practice, until your schedule becomes full.

Finally, there are some suggestions that will require you to prove that you have longevity before they will become available. These fall into two groups: professional exposure and community exposure. Hopefully you will take away some ideas that will quickly rocket you from relative obscurity to the celebrated new surgeon in town.

J. D. Paletta, MD, FACS
The Georgia Institute for Plastic Surgery, Savannah, GA, USA

Cold Call Visits to Referring Doctors

When you arrive in your new practice, whether you are joining an existing practice or starting out solo, you will not be immediately busy. Don't let this worry you—it will come soon enough! From a clinical perspective, you might find that you are the busiest after typical working hours and have more free time than you are accustomed to during daylight. In this early phase of your practice, spend time learning from your partners or other senior surgeons in town. Take advantage of the free time during the day to meet your colleagues.

Compile lists of specialties that will be likely to refer to you. For instance, plastic surgery and dermatology, vascular surgery and nephrology, cardiac surgery and cardiology, general surgery and gastroenterology, etc. Locate the offices of the specialties that go hand in hand with your own, and visit them! A personal introduction will go a long way, and being able to connect a friendly face to a name will win you referrals in no time. You do not necessarily need an appointment, but you should be prepared. Before you arrive, have business cards and, if possible, brochures available to leave so that they can easily remember you and give something to patients who will need to contact and find your office. When you arrive at the office, give the receptionist your card, and let them know that you would love to meet with Dr. X to introduce yourself. It is exceedingly unusual that they will not take a few minutes to meet you, schedule permitting.

When you meet, ask questions to determine how you could be helpful to their practice. That may include how to make referrals to you easier or the types of patients that may need your help managing. Early on, these referrals may be small cases, undesirable cases, or even difficult patients. Take these referrals very seriously and manage them with care. Chances are your referring doctor is testing you to see if they can depend on you to take care of their patients. Make it a point to follow up, and continue to express your interest in receiving their referrals. They will appreciate your hard work, and it will pay off in no time.

Eat Breakfast or Lunch in the Hospital and Network with the Physicians

In addition to visiting potential referring physicians in their offices, make it a point to eat breakfast and lunch at the hospital everyday. If your hospital has a physician's lounge/cafeteria and provides a free meal, I can assure you that they will be busy! You will find new members of the medical staff who, like you, will not be very busy but can grow to become excellent referral sources as both of your careers grow.

You will also find senior members of the medical staff who might be looking for someone to refer challenging cases to, or perhaps the doctor they referred to has retired. Hidden opportunities can only reveal themselves if you go looking for them! This will be a rare opportunity to take a true lunch hour or longer. In fact, it is not out of the question to have lunch with a group, round on a patient or two, and then return to have a drink with another group! The more groups you introduce yourself to, the wider your referring base will become.

Assist with Cases of Other Surgeons

You can also be productive during the day while expanding your education and generating income. The best way to do this is to make yourself available to your partners as an assistant. Not only will you have the potential to learn something, but you will effectively lighten their load, show that you are a team player, and make a little income all at the same time!

If you do not have partners, ask other surgeons in town if they are in need of an assistant on any upcoming cases. This will also help them to get to know you better and give them a comfort level about your skill set. Lastly, if they do not need an assistant, perhaps you can observe and learn tips and tricks for handling different situations that may arise. Reaching out to other surgeons in town will help you become a known entity and build relationships so that you can call on them when you need a hand.

Taking Call

The bulk of your work will not magically appear between the hours of 9:00 am and 5:00 pm. The largest source of referrals will come from being on call. Take as much call as you feel comfortable with. You may even want to solicit extra call from your partners or other physicians in town. The more you are available, the faster your practice will grow, and you will eventually be able to taper off the extra call.

Be careful to avoid burnout from overworking yourself as you begin to establish your practice—this is a marathon, not a sprint. If you are tired and overworked, it is more likely that you will not be as pleasant to patients and staff! Every interaction you have with a patient and/or hospital staff member is a potential referral source for the future. For obvious reasons, the operating room staff would refer patients to a surgeon who is not necessarily the best technical surgeon but the surgeon who treats them with kindness and respect and who is technically adequate. There is nothing wrong with being known as the nice guy!

Professional Exposure

Professional exposure consists of activities that are designed to introduce you to other physicians, either initially or repeatedly. The simplest thing to do is to attend medical staff meeting and local medical society meetings. Medical staff meeting used to be mandatory and, therefore, were well attended. Even if they are not mandatory, it is still a good idea to attend a few and determine if this is a worthwhile use of your time. Included in medical staff meeting are departmental meetings. Medical staff and medical societies will typically have social events or outings that are an excellent way to meet physicians and their families in a more casual setting. Becoming friends with colleagues never hurts the referral process and will help you to become settled in your new environment.

As you become more established, you may want to consider expanding your involvement in hospital politics, such as the medical staff or hospital committees. Not only will this expose you to the leadership of the hospital, but also involvement in some committees will affect your practice, such as in the assigning of block time.

Community Exposure

Community exposure is designed to introduce you directly to patients. Some of these opportunities are within the hospital, such as seeing patients in the wound center or hyperbaric oxygen chamber. If these opportunities are available, seek them out when you are less busy, and as your practice grows, you can decrease or eliminate your involvement as necessary.

Outside of the hospital, there may arise the chance to be involved in health screening for skin cancer, vascular disease, or colorectal cancer, just to name a few. Additionally, there may be community organizations or corporations that would welcome a physician to come and speak during one of their group meetings. Remember to tailor your talk to the group that will be attending in terms of age and gender. Making yourself available in a setting that is familiar to them will encourage them to reach out when they need your help.

There will also be opportunities that do not require medical skill at all. They include leadership groups, young professional associations, ethnic societies, and sporting groups in your area. Involvement in these types of organizations will obviously be based on your available time and interest in the group. Sponsoring local charity events and youth sporting teams helps to get your name out into the community. Find something that you are passionate about, and volunteer your time and, when possible, your financial resources. It may help your practice, but more importantly, it will afford you an excellent opportunity to get involved in your community, build lasting relationships, and maybe even have a little fun!

Going the Extra Mile for Great Customer Service

You have worked hard to foster relationships with physicians in your area and get patients to your office. Now you have to continue to work hard to get them to come back and, more importantly, to refer friends and family to you! Part of this is managing your online reputation, and you must provide excellent customer service with every patient or referring doctor interaction. Dropping the ball even one time can damage your reputation and undo months of groundwork that went into building the relationship.

Great customer service starts with an easily accessible office, with ample parking, and continues with a tasteful reception area. Your staff should be professional, polite, and welcoming. You should provide prompt and comprehensive communication with referring physicians. After same-day surgery or procedures, make it a point to personally call the patients to check in on them or deliver pathology reports. They appreciate your extra efforts, and they will tell their friends. Doing the little things that are not medically necessary to provide great care are what sets apart a mediocre practice from a great practice with excellent customer service.

Chapter 41
When Your Patient Dies

Marc Neff

We became surgeons to help people and to heal people, through long hours of honing our craft spent in an 18 by 18 foot sterile room. We practice perfection every single day. It's what our patients expect and what we demand of ourselves. Many of my residents and students will hear my voice in their heads years later saying sternly, "The only part of the operation that the patient sees are the incisions. Make sure they are perfect." That is why we take complications so devastatingly. And why, when our patient dies, we often find ourselves lost. There is an emotional part to this and then a practical part.

Sad but true, not every patient has a surgical problem we can fix. We didn't cause the perforated colon cancer metastatic to the liver in the 37-year-olds. We didn't cause the intractable abdominal pain in the Crohn's patient with ten different operations. And we certainly aren't responsible when our patient comes into the trauma bay pulseless with a penetrating gunshot wound to the chest. But, in the end, we do feel a certainly amount of responsibility that maybe their death is on us. Why?

As surgeons, we are born problem solvers. We think that every patient is a complicated multiple-choice question after years of standardized testing. Every problem has a correct answer. The problem with that upbringing is that for many patients, the answer of death isn't an acceptable one. We blame ourselves for not studying hard enough, for not scrubbing in the OR enough, and for not checking every laboratory value, progress note, and diagnostic study with the radiologist ourselves.

There is a normal reaction to death we are taught in medical school, anger, fear, frustration, anxiety, depression, or acceptance. This is what we are taught. Sadly, we aren't taught that these stages don't have to come in any particular order. We aren't taught that you can spend different amounts of time in each stage. And certainly we are never taught that you can get lost in a stage forever. This reaction to death is what families go through, and what we go through to some degree, as physicians.

M. Neff, MD, FACS, FASMBS
Center for Surgical Weight Loss, Jefferson Health New Jersey, Cherry Hill, NJ, USA

© Springer International Publishing AG, part of Springer Nature 2018
K. Yoon-Flannery et al. (eds.), *A Surgeon's Path*,
https://doi.org/10.1007/978-3-319-78846-3_41

But, while the emotional side of losing a patient is an important one and one that is mentioned first to highlight its importance, there are at least two others that deserve mention and that are on the more practical side.

Firstly, when your patient dies, you need to pull together your emotions and talk with the family. Recognize that what you say may take only a few minutes, but it is something that every family member there will remember for the rest of their lives. Be sincere and patient and honest. Sit down. Have your staff take the family to a quiet and private area. Alert the chaplain if you haven't already and security if there are too many people or you get a vibe that they may be emotionally out of control or violent. At this point, the family has become your patient. Your sensitivity here is what they will remember or, lack of it, what they will never forget. I find that the best thing to do is to get close to the family. Summarize what happened. Don't waste words and beat around the bush. Be succinct. Also, emphasize that you did everything that you could. Emphasize that they didn't suffer. Have the nurses clean up the room and the body, and make the room peaceful. Give the family time to say their goodbyes.

Second, when your patient dies, you will have some business to take care of. I mention this last, because it is sometimes a needless distraction while everyone is trying to process, but it is nonetheless very real. Your hospital will have policies about filling out the death certificate, on what to do with the funeral home, and in regard to a possible transplant status. Follow the nurse's lead. They will guide you. You also have to alert your partners and your malpractice carrier if you have any suspicion at all that a potential claim may be filed. It seems dirty to do this, but it's very real and necessary. What happens when patient of yours dies may sadly be a lawsuit, and you have to prepare yourself for that possibility.

Chapter 42
Innovation

John R. Bookwalter

Introduction

Each of us has an occasional good idea about how to improve some activity in our personal or professional life. We can change the way we do something to see how it works out and then decide whether or not to incorporate it into our routine. There is no need for copyrights, patents, or licenses to move forward. If, on the other hand, we feel that an idea may have some commercial value, we have to move forward in a different way.

Commercialization and Protection of Intellectual Property

At some point we have to protect our ideas from encroachment or theft. We can apply for a patent, which can be very expensive and expires in 17 years or a copyright, which does not expire but insures that no one can call a similar device by the same name.

In my own experience, patents are best applied for when the product development phase is well under way, with the inventors as co-applicants along with the manufacturer and a co-developer. Following this course of action for success means that the inventor becomes part of a team, and, as with any successful team, it is critical to (1) have confidence in the integrity of the people you are working with and (2) to treat the members of your team with respect. In this way you will not waste money (as I have done) on ideas that don't pan out.

J. R. Bookwalter, MD, FACS
Brattleboro Memorial Hospital, Brattleboro, VT, USA

Product Development and Improvement

The best situation is to work with a company that manufactures and sells products similar to what you are trying to develop. There is no substitute for this process of prototyping, trial and evaluation, followed by improvement of the prototype until the team feels that the product will be commercially viable. To be commercially viable, the product must be cost-effective. It must simplify or replace a function in a way that saves the customer time and/or money. The more experiences that the team has and the more mutual respect among team members, the smoother this process will be.

Production

Ideally, production should be as close to the product development facility as possible, so that improvements can be made based on customer feedback. When production of the Bookwalter Retractor was shifted to Germany and I was prevented from interacting directly with them, a few products were introduced with my name on them that I felt were not very good from an ergonomic standpoint.

Sales and Marketing

It is important to have a good relationship with the Sales and Marketing group because they work directly with the customers and they have such a challenging job in today's medical environment. Treating these folks with respect and listening to their feedback can be extremely valuable in finding ways to improve the product. From their ranks have come some of my best friends.

Finally, a few maxims to keep in mind going forward include:

1. Good judgment comes from experience and experience comes from bad judgment.
2. No project succeeds without some failure and revision along the way.

Compensation

If you are going to form a company and devote full time to an idea, you will probably have to find some investor whom you can persuade to help you going forward. This approach carries greater risk but also, if successful, great rewards.

On the other hand, if you are going to license the idea to someone else, it is important to have a relationship of mutual trust and respect. Royalties can run in the range of around 5% for patented ideas and around 3% for non-patented items and are negotiable.

Chapter 43
Future Technology in Healthcare

Robert Neff

Introduction

As I write this chapter during my travels back from a conference in New York City on healthcare technology, I realize how easy it is to forget how many forms of technoloy (digital, devices, pharmaceutical) are all working to improve health. I live much of my life reviewing digital technologies and systems that improve the delivery and operations of healthcare. In this chapter we will discuss many areas of digital technology.

Medical Devices

The term "medical device" can be quite broad and widely ranging. Technically pacemakers and tongue depressors are both medical devices (granted one is a Class I device and the other pacemaker is a Class III). The number of medical devices that are being created today is staggering. Advances in product development across all industries have allowed new devices to be created even by start-up companies.

Additionally, foundations like the XPRIZE which recently sponsored a contest to build a medical tricorder (similar to what was shown in Star Trek) have spurred innovation. All of this innovation means that beyond the traditional crop of physiological monitors, ventilators, and infusion pumps, there are a lot of new devices that are becoming available in every area from monitoring to intervention to a combination of the two. This area of development is projected to continue to explode, and new medical devices will gain traction in health systems.

R. Neff, BSc
Digital Innovation and Consumer Experience Group (DICE),
Thomas Jefferson University and Jefferson Health,
Philadelphia, PA, USA
e-mail: robert.neff@jefferson.edu

© Springer International Publishing AG, part of Springer Nature 2018
K. Yoon-Flannery et al. (eds.), *A Surgeon's Path*,
https://doi.org/10.1007/978-3-319-78846-3_43

Consumer-Grade Medical Devices

Consumer-grade medical devices are an interesting concept because they bring technology directly to a consumer in their home. Monitoring blood glucose levels, checking heart rate, and many other types of monitoring can now easily be done at home. This provides a challenge but also great opportunity. There is currently an important question about what to do with all of the data from consumer medical devices, which is often known as "patient-generated health data." It is an important question, because data from these devices might not be quite as accurate due to the quality of the devices or the fact that the operator of the device (the patient) may not be properly trained on how to use it to collect the data correctly. Despite the temptation to ignore these devices, it is critical to understand how to leverage data from this crop of new technology. As the capabilities of these devices will continue to expand, the patients will expect providers to know what to do with their data.

Digital Technologies

By far the largest group of technology in this category is mobile applications. Mobile apps range from technologies that are as basic as medication reminder apps to systems that include telehealth to the much more extreme, such as those utilizing accelerometers and other sensors to collect data for clinical trials. The benefit of mobile apps and their proliferation is that they greatly increase access and remove barriers for much of the public. The challenge is that this technology is evolving incredibly quickly while not necessarily being validated as compared to traditional healthcare technology. In addition to mobile apps, online patient portals, quick patient registration and scheduling systems are also gaining in use. Perhaps one of the most interesting impacts of this technology is what is often referred to as "physician transparency"—the ability for patients to see reviews and even star ratings for their providers—similar to how they shop for other services online. These tools, which increase the knowledge of patients as consumers in healthcare, will start to drive competition among healthcare providers and hopefully drive the industry to ultimately provide better healthcare and patient experiences.

Genomics, Personalized Medicine, and Pharmaceuticals

As technology continues to improve in the area of genome mapping, we are starting to see many more products aimed at providing personalized healthcare. The technology that exists to analyze data on a large scale (often known as *big data*) is improving exponentially. This means data analysis that was very lengthy and costly is now becoming quicker and less expensive. In addition, the automation of data analysis available now allows chemical compounds as well as physical parts (e.g., scaffolding for tissue growth, etc.) to be created automatically based on customized analysis of a person's DNA. We are quickly approaching a world where the medicine will be completely customized to a specific individual based on their DNA.

The examples of technology shared here are specific examples and not meant to be a survey of the entire industry of new technology in healthcare. These are just a few of the examples of how new technology will change healthcare. The way we think of healthcare will change thanks to technology. Healthcare will continue to evolve to focus more on personalized care with a physician helping as a consultant based on all the information gathered from sensors and systems monitoring your health. Physicians will likely focus primarily on acute issues that arise unexpectedly—after all, without cancer, viruses, and hereditary diseases, they should have a lot of time freed up.

Chapter 44
Interacting with Residents

Sandra R. DiBrito and Elliott R. Haut

Introduction

Working with residents can be rewarding, adding meaning and value to everyday work. Unfortunately, it can also seem cumbersome, intimidating, or overwhelming to attendings who are trying to get their feet on the ground in a new position. The key to developing an excellent working relationship with residents is establishing mutual respect. Here, we discuss some ways you can gain and maintain respect and offer some common pitfalls to avoid.

Respect

First and foremost, remember that you were once a resident too, perhaps not long ago, and that you also struggled through your first incisions, sutures, and mistakes. Allow yourself to appreciate the time and energy it took for you to develop into the competent and confident surgeon that you are, and practice self-respect by focusing on cultivating that further as you begin your practice as an attending. It is imperative that you demonstrate confidence in the operating room. You are the attending,

S. R. DiBrito, MD
Department of General Surgery, Johns Hopkins University School of Medicine,
Baltimore, MD, USA
e-mail: sdibrito@jhmi.edu

E. R. Haut, MD, PhD, FACS
Division of Trauma Surgery and Critical Care, Department of Surgery,
Johns Hopkins University School of Medicine, Baltimore, MD, USA
e-mail: ehaut1@jhmi.edu

© Springer International Publishing AG, part of Springer Nature 2018
K. Yoon-Flannery et al. (eds.), *A Surgeon's Path*,
https://doi.org/10.1007/978-3-319-78846-3_44

calling the shots and making decisions. Even if you are not certain of the next move, or the situation is getting more intense than anticipated, be confident in your training and your skills. It is appropriate to share with the residents that you might feel uncertain about the next move. Even though admitting your limitations seems intimidating, or that it makes you appear weak, residents benefit from learning about how to handle difficult situations and proceed safely. Watching an attending decide to ask for help, take a moment and review imaging, or discuss aloud the alternate approaches gives the resident a valuable learning experience. On the other hand, don't make the resident feel they need to be the decision-maker to avoid disaster. This shakes their confidence in you and will erode their respect for you as a leader and mentor.

Garnering respect from residents means that you stick to a high standard of care for your patients. Be clear and concise in your directions when residents ask your preferences, and try to maintain a predictable pattern of behavior. This is good practice overall, as it helps hone your attending "style" and helps residents understand how to care for your patients. If you are perceived as demanding, this is a backhanded compliment; it suggests that the residents feel they need to work hard and provide a high standard of care for your patients. As much as residents need autonomy to develop their clinical and decision-making skills, they also need discipline and structure to feel safe making those smaller decisions, knowing that you will be there to back them up if a decision turns out to be less than ideal.

Autonomy

Autonomy is another way attendings can show respect for their residents. Despite the fact that you have many more years of training than your trainees, it is important to cultivate a sense of respect and collegiality, seeing patient care as a team sport with many participants. When residents feel that their time, energy, and ideas are respected, they are often willing to work harder and take constructive suggestions for improvement. This does not mean you need to actually carry out all of the suggestions of your residents, but allowing them to develop plans, encouraging them to take the next step, and even letting them fail by virtue of following through with their own decisions can be a valuable teaching strategy. If residents are too paralyzed by fear or shame to make decisions around small details of patient care, they will never develop the confidence needed to perform as attendings in the future. Much of residency is learning behaviors of a variety of attendings, emulating these behaviors, and ultimately taking parts and pieces from each teacher. Ultimately, all attendings are just an amalgam of their influences, and you have the power to shape the next generation of surgeons just by leading by example. Choose to be a positive role model, rather than the ones they learn not to be like.

Education

If you are at an academic institution, you are probably expected to perform some resident education. This can be perceived in many ways—as a burden, a chore, or an opportunity for personal growth—the choice is yours. There is nothing more demoralizing to residents than trying to learn from an attending who clearly does not value teaching. This can be communicated openly ("Well, I am contractually obligated to give you a lecture this morning"), somewhat openly ("They just don't pay me enough to teach these labs – I need to be in the operating room hitting my RVU target!"), or subtly, manifested by showing up late, unprepared, or unengaged. While performing teaching duties may be part of your contract, taking away from operating room time, and requires preparation that you might not have time to perform, in order to maintain a good working relationship with residents, it is important that you keep these sentiments to yourself.

When you have to give a lecture or lab, focus on the task at hand. Show up prepared, even if you only have a few minutes to review the topic. Look at an old PowerPoint slide deck or glance at the latest review article on the subject. Even 5 minutes of preparation is better than showing up late and asking aloud "What is this lecture supposed to be about?" When attendings show up unprepared, residents feel like a burden to the department and lose respect for the teacher. It is rightly perceived as hypocritical to expect residents to show up to a surgical case fully prepared, having researched the patient and operation ahead of time, while not demonstrating that same degree of preparation as an attending.

Most surgeons are busy building a practice, managing patients, and trying to balance life at work and home. You may feel you are "too busy to teach." Fortunately, there is no such thing as "too busy to teach" if you know how to teach in a few different ways. Formal PowerPoint presentations and "chalk talks" are great ways to educate residents. However, some of the most valuable teaching happens informally during your everyday practice. Just vocalizing your thought process while making surgical decisions, either in the operating room or in clinic, is valuable teaching. Verbalizing steps of an operation, describing anatomical landmarks that you are trying to find (or avoid!), and discussing instrument choices are all things that can be done in the moment in an operating room, do not require extra time to prepare, and will win respect and appreciation from residents. Describing these things may not be easy when your mind is busy focusing on the task at hand, and this style of teaching takes some work to perfect, but is worth practicing for the sake of building your reputation as a great teacher among residents. Mentioning recent review articles, guidelines, or websites can also guide residents to high-yield, information-packed resources.

Personas to Avoid

Maintaining a professional relationship with your colleagues and residents is an important part of establishing yourself as a respected attending in your hospital and department. Unfortunately, there are many ways to compromise this relationship that can permanently tarnish your reputation. Here we discuss common pitfalls of different attending personas, how they can be harmful, and how to avoid them.

"Best Friend"

The attending "best friend" is someone who builds friendships with residents, as opposed to professional, mutually respectful working relationships. Being kind and cordial to residents is an asset, and being friendly is welcome. However, some attendings take this too far and end up blurring the lines of the hierarchy. Examples of this behavior include frequently going out with residents to restaurants, bars, or clubs, giving residents gifts, or going out of your way to spend free time with residents in a social setting. These seemingly harmless activities may make you feel like the life of the party, but they can also erode the respect that you are trying to establish as a new attending. To be perceived as a leader and mentor, it is best to avoid this type of behavior. Being kind, taking your team out for a round of drinks after a rotation, and saying "happy birthday" to residents are appropriate ways to show your appreciation. Drawing the line between "friend" and "colleague" is imperative for success.

"Over-Sharer"

When in the operating room, there is often time for small talk and frequently long discussions. In addition to avoiding politics, it is important to decide your boundaries when sharing information about your personal and family life. How much you share (or choose not to share) is closely noted by residents, and what one person might find reasonable, another may find totally inappropriate for discussing in the workplace. Additionally, residents don't always feel comfortable sharing details of their personal lives. You should create a safe, cordial environment in your operating room, and shouldn't make assumptions about what you expect to hear about a resident's social situation. You are in charge of your operating room and, with that, in charge of setting your own limits. Be aware that while trying to focus on the operation, most residents don't need to hear every detail of your family's summer vacation, and many might not feel comfortable divulging details about their off time to you.

"Town Gossip"

To fill the silence during cases or between patients in clinic, it may be tempting to talk about the latest departmental gossip. This is an easy way to become the informant of the entire residency when it comes to matters that should generally be kept behind closed doors or at a senior level. Seemingly harmless gossip can quickly snowball into accusations about colleagues in your department that could be damaging to their reputation or the entire department. Discussing who might be looking elsewhere for a new position, who is unsatisfied in their current role, and who feels a certain way about interacting with residents can lead to unintended consequences and could compromise your colleagues. Attendings must set an example for behavior, and badmouthing the decision-making, surgical skills, or patient outcomes of your colleagues cultivates a sense of distrust and disrespect in your department. This will make residents feel less secure in their own decision-making and skill development and stifles their growth in the long run. Respecting your peers by keeping conversation positive can help maintain a strong network of trust. The best rule of thumb is to keep your opinions to yourself and keep the operating room talk to either surgery or the music choice in the room.

"Guilt-Tripper"

As patient care becomes more complex and multidisciplinary, residents are performing different duties than were expected 5 or 10 years ago. With that in mind, try to respect the evolution of training and what it means for residents. There is nothing worse than working to the point of physical and mental exhaustion, only to be taunted for not working long or hard enough. While we are all aware of restrictions placed on duty hours, everyone should also appreciate that 80-hours weeks do not reflect the entire amount of time that residents spend working, either in-house or from home. It does not garner respect to deride residents for ONLY working 80 hours when you used to work 110 hours. The fact of the matter is turnover in hospitals is higher than ever, patients are living longer with more complex diseases, and surgical science is developing so quickly that it is nearly impossible to keep up with the latest treatments and therapies available for every specialty. Being in-house every other night and in charge of 100 patients for 110 hours per week for 5 years might have been your experience as a resident, but reiterating this over and over makes you sound like a parent who walked uphill both ways to school through the snow every day during their entire childhood. Making residents feel guilty for duty hour restrictions is demoralizing and unhelpful. The easiest way to address work hours is to encourage compliance and leave the specifics to the program directors and coordinators.

"My Way"

Everyone has their own technique, approach, and style when caring for patients both in and out of the operating room. Whether starting subcutaneous heparin, pulling nasogastric tubes, removing Foley catheters, or advancing diets, residents are aware that every attending likes it "their way." It is unhelpful to reiterate phrases like "This isn't my way, it's the RIGHT way," because there is definitely more than one way to successfully care for patients in almost every clinical scenario. Running or interrupted midline closure? Subcuticular sutures with or without knots? Glue or gauze? If there are data to support your practice, provide it. Seemingly small details make up your "style." Residents will respect your style, but to be successful in achieving the detailed care you intend for your patient, be consistent. If your style is predictable, residents can learn the logic behind your choices and will do their best to fall in line. Avoid phrases using the word "always" when describing how a procedure should be done, because it is likely that many of your colleagues do things just a little differently. Also, avoid repeatedly using the phrases "When I was in training, we always…." and "The only way to…." Generally speaking, it goes without saying that the way you operate or care for patients comes from your experience in training. No need to harp on this every time. There is no need to insinuate that where you came from routinely did something better than where you are now. To residents, this behavior is the attending equivalent of a resident repeatedly telling you how your colleagues do things differently when they are questioning your decisions. These behaviors convey insecurity, which does not build respect. Instead, you should own your decisions and be consistent.

The Successful Mentor

While there are seemingly infinite ways to flounder in the development and maintenance of working relationships with residents, the recipe for success can be boiled down to a few simple points. Here, we present a list of the top ten ways an attending can achieve excellent interactions with residents. Be careful; as you put these tips into practice, residents may begin to orbit you more closely and see you as a mentor. This transition, from attending to official mentor, takes time and effort to develop, but will pay dividends in a lifelong career. You begin by guiding trainees through an exceedingly difficult phase of their career and end up with well-trained, respectful, and appreciative young colleagues who will inevitably disperse to other institutions across the country and carry on your wisdom to the next generation.

Top Ten Qualities of Attendings (From a Resident Perspective)

1. *Honesty*—Being honest with patients, colleagues, and trainees is noted, appreciated, and respected. Being honest can be painful at times (when breaking bad news to a patient, admitting an error at morbidity and mortality conference (M&M), or giving constructive feedback to a struggling resident), but earning a reputation as an honest attending is invaluable.
2. *Respect*—Respecting each member of the surgical team allows the team to function optimally. Respect people's time, energy, and humanity, and you will be miles ahead of the game.
3. *Confidence*—Have confidence in yourself, so residents can have confidence in you too! You completed years of training, and your experience is increasing exponentially. Lean on that body of experience and build your confidence, at the bedside and in the operating room, to help build your relationship with residents.
4. *Listens*—If you pay attention to your resident while they are talking to you, it will repay you tenfold. Not only are they occasionally telling you important clinical details but also feeling like they have your attention comes across as respectful and will build your rapport with residents. Put your phone in your pocket and make eye contact—it goes a long way.
5. *Team player*—As the attending, you are the team leader; you set the tone for the group. Visit your residents on their turf and on the wards, and see patients together. Treating the hospital and operating room like a shared environment helps everyone on the team feel included, which results in improved morale. Use "we should" not "you should" when talking about patient care.
6. *Human*—Don't pretend you aren't tired or hungry too. Knowing that you are human and that you actually don't want to spend 100% of your waking moments in the hospital makes you relatable, believable, and more trustworthy. You don't have to talk about your family or home life all the time, but admitting you have more in your life than surgery is reassuring.
7. *Knowledgeable*—Keeping up on the literature is good for you, your patients, and your residents. Being aware of a new trial or discussing a review article or guideline encourages residents to keep reading and builds their trust in you as a knowledgeable entity.
8. *Present*—Attend department events, show up for conferences, and be a presence in the hospital. Put in face time with your patients and team. It is hard to look up to someone who is never around.
9. *Supportive*—If residents know you are there to help them back up after they fall flat on their face, they will be more willing to go out on a limb for you. This means supporting them in the operating room as they are employing new techniques or backing them up at M&M as they defend your mistakes.

10. *Raise the bar*—Residents want to improve and become the best surgeon they can possibly be. Setting high standards conveys that you have the best interest of your residents at heart. If you expect your residents to perform well, they probably will. If you expect them to fail, that is almost a guarantee.

Conclusion

Working at an academic institution has both perks and drawbacks, and working with residents can fall into either category depending on your perception. At the end of the day, residents are working hard to provide the best patient care possible while learning enough to become a successful attending in a very short time. Treating them with respect will help you develop the best working relationship possible, and behaving in a way that commands their respect will ultimately result in optimal care for your patients.

Suggested Reading

Lee A, Dennis C, Campbell P. Nature's guide for mentors. *Nature*. 2007;447:791–7.
Souba WW. Mentoring young academic surgeons, our most precious asset. J Surg Res. 1999; 82(2):113–20.
Vaughn V, Saint S, Chopra V. Mentee missteps: tales from the academic trenches. JAMA. 2017; 317(5):475–6.

Chapter 45
Professionalism

Linda Szczurek

Professionalism is a concept that is rarely formally taught but is the most important component of your entire career because it applies to everything you do as a physician. Despite the changes in today's culture (and the way you may be treated sometimes), doctors are still highly regarded by society and the community and are held to higher standards compared to many other jobs. There are few trades where you are "expected" to do everything in your power for the better of society and patients regardless of how you are treated, monetary gain, or other burdens that are placed on your life.

Learning professionalism as a doctor is a skill that is acquired over time during our training and through experience. Whether or not you realized it at the time, your first step in professionalism was taking the Hippocratic Oath during your White Coat Ceremony on the first day of medical school. Professionalism is not black and white. It is a spectrum composed of many different parts. A person can be great at some of the aspects such as treating others with respect but awful at timeliness and always running late in office hours or arrival to the OR. In this chapter, we will review the key components that make up professionalism and some obvious and not so obvious tips to hone your skills.

In 2002, the American Board of Internal Medicine Foundation, the American College of Physicians, and the European Federation of Internal Medicine published Medical Professionalism in the New Millennium: A Physician Charter. The fundamental principles of the charter include patient welfare, patient altruism, and social justice. Since first released, the charter has been endorsed by more than 130 organizations. These three key components all focus on placing the patient above all else. As physicians, we are obligated to look after patient's best interests, treating them to the best of our abilities despite the patient's class, race, or insurance status.

L. Szczurek, DO, FACOS
Jefferson Health New Jersey, Cherry Hill, NJ, USA

© Springer International Publishing AG, part of Springer Nature 2018
K. Yoon-Flannery et al. (eds.), *A Surgeon's Path*,
https://doi.org/10.1007/978-3-319-78846-3_45

This seems ingrained in most doctors from day one since the main reason that we choose our profession was to be able to help people. However, as your training and experience progressed, you probably realized that it is not always that easy. Yes, none of us would ever do anything to harm a patient intentionally, but do we always and can we always do what is best? There will be days when you explain to a patient that you are trying to help and review what needs to be done to make them better, but no matter how hard you try, the patient does not want to listen, and they leave the office or sign out of the hospital against medical advice. Another example involves dealing with insurance companies. In today's cost-conscious healthcare environment, it can be very difficult to obtain insurance pre-certification or pre-authorization for certain tests or procedures. You know the test or surgery that you ordered for your patient is the right thing, but no matter how much you advocate for your patient and argue with the random insurance guy on the other end of the telephone, that guy just won't budge, and now the patient has to suffer the consequences, or you have to compromise care and change your plan to something that may not be as good. I spend a portion of my time at a "clinic" working with patients who are uninsured or underinsured on a regular basis, and I find this to be one of the most difficult aspects of my job. The patient needs help but cannot get it because of lack of coverage. I cannot even tell you how many women I have seen over the past few years who present with large breast cancers because they did not have insurance and could not get access to a mammogram sooner even though they knew there was a problem. Unfortunately, this is a society issue that needs resolution on a global scale. I have learned to accept the struggle one patient at a time doing what I can for that individual and not getting frustrated by the process. Patient advocacy is only one piece of professionalism and below I will touch on others.

Expertise in Your Field

As a doctor, you pledge to maintain a certain level of proficiency in your field. After training is completed, this will fall into your lap. Although all specialties have some sort of maintenance of certification requirements and states have licensure requirements, it will be up to you to keep up with new technology, techniques, and standards. You will no longer have a program director telling you what you need to learn. You will have to seek out conferences, journals, and other sources of continuing medical education (CME) in order to practice at the highest level possible.

High Standards, Accountability, and Responsibility

These tie closely with expertise in your field. Again, you are now responsible for maintaining your top-notch skills and knowledge. You need to actively read the newest journal articles in your field and search out CME activities to further your education as medicine and medical technology are constantly evolving. In addition, you will have a ton of paperwork to keep up with. There is an endless stream of dictations and notes from your hospital patients, residents' orders and notes to sign off on and electronic medical record notes and test results to complete from your office. The hospital where you work at if you are in private practice or the hospital you are employed by will track the completion of all this mandatory paperwork as a quality measure. If you do not stay on top of these responsibilities in a timely manner, when collecting a bonus or renewing your contract comes, this may impact you negatively. Medicare and other insurance companies are also scrutinizing quality and standards, and there is currently a shift of payments and reimbursements based on these measures that you will be held accountable for. More importantly, your paperwork does need to be finished as soon as possible because it can affect patient care. For example, you partner sees a patient in the office for a procedure this week, and the patient has a problem so is back to see you in 2 days because your partner is not available. If he did not complete his office note, you will not be very happy when you cannot figure out exactly what was done or discussed.

Respect for Yourself and Others

The best way to earn respect is to treat others with respect. You need to be kind and courteous to everyone around you including your colleagues, staff, and patients. In the hospital and office, one of the best ways to show respect to your patients and their families is to listen carefully to everything they have to say without cutting them off. We are often rushing because we are busy, and it is easy to interrupt trying to speed things along. Listening is also very important in the OR. For example, everyone including you should be quiet and paying attention during the "time-out" prior to surgery as this has been proven to prevent medical errors.

Timeliness

With our hectic schedules of office hours and operating room cases, some days it will be impossible to stay on time with everything. I already discussed the importance of completion of paperwork on time in the accountability section above. Many hospitals/operating rooms will mandate that you be on time for your scheduled cases especially if it is the first case of the day to prevent backup throughout the rest of the day. At the hospital where I work, you must show up before 7:15 am for a 7:30 am start time. If you are consistently late, you will have your morning block time taken away. The on time first start measure is also viewed as a quality measure that can be tied to compensation. Staying on time with office hours is always a challenge. It does get easier with experience because you can judge how long certain appointments will take. No one likes to sit in the waiting room for an hour to see the doctor, so try your best to keep the day moving. You should not rush patients out, but if you are running late, the patients appreciate it if you apologize or explain why they had to wait.

Honesty/Integrity/Confidentiality/Ethics

These items will play a significant role in your everyday interactions with patients. In today's medical legal environment, there is a strong emphasis on patient confidentiality and HIPAA. You should not be sharing patients' medical information with anyone who is not involved in taking care of the patient, and you should always remember to ask the patient if you may talk about his or her care with family or friends. Reported HIPAA violations can lead to hefty fines. Surgeons love to operate but not all patients should have or need an operation. We frequently run into family members who want everything done for mom or dad who is 95 years old with a tracheostomy, feeding tube, and no quality of life. In this event, it is our job to explain to the patient and family that the patient has an overall poor prognosis and will likely suffer rather than benefit from any major surgical intervention. Another example that commonly occurs is a patient pushing for surgery for abdominal pain or some other issues with a completely negative work-up. If you find yourself backed into a corner and you do not believe an operation will help a patient, you can always tell the patient no and send the individual to another surgeon for a second opinion. Letting someone talk to you into something that you do not feel is in the best interest of the patient will never end well. You cannot be sued for recommending a second opinion. Being honest with patients and families is essential to professionalism especially when there is a complication or mistake. Trying to lie or cover up a problem will only lead to bigger issues down the road if you have to sit in front of a judge and a jury. The majority of medical legal research shows that patients and families understand that there are risks involved in medical care and that no doctor is perfect. They are much more likely to respond in a non-litigious manner when you are up-front and honest and apologize sincerely.

Maintaining Composure Under Stress/Conduct/ Reaction to Mistake

Professionalism does not mean perfectionism. At some point relatively soon, you will find yourself in a difficult situation. It could be a very tough case, a patient or family that is hard to deal with or a patient complication, and you must maintain your strength, composure, and confidence. I remember a specific attending during my training that was easily rattled in the operating room every time there was a small bump in the road. He would start yelling at the nurse and scrub technicians and even throw instruments across the room. I learned to duck quickly and also that I never wanted to be the "surgeon" that the staff never wants to work with and talks about his childish behavior behind his back. I also remember 1 day while working with a resident when the clip from the cystic artery fell off and blood started spraying all over (it always looks a lot worse than it is due to the magnificent of the laparoscopic equipment). I did not yell or scream or kick the resident out of the way. I calmly told the resident what to do and let the resident fix the issue placing new clips on the bleeding artery. The rest of the case went smoothly, and at the end, the resident came up to me and thanked me and told me she was very impressed with how I handled the situation.

Appearance

The operating room is a great place to work because we basically get to wear pajamas most of the day. Do not get carried away making scrubs your everyday attire. If you are wearing scrubs in the operating room or making rounds on the floors, make sure they are clean and that you are wearing your clean white coat as well. For office hours and meetings, business attire is appropriate. We all look a little disheveled after a bad night on call, but do your best to look clean and professional on a regular basis.

Suggested Reading

American Board of Internal Medicine Foundation. American College of Physicians–American Society of Internal Medicine Foundation. European Federation of Internal Medicine Medical professionalism in the new millennium: a physician charter. Ann Intern Med. 2002;136(3):243–6.

Chapter 46
Research

Fabian M. Johnston and Elliott R. Haut

Introduction

Congratulations! You have finished your residency/fellowship and completed the culmination of 5–10 years of hard work. As you read this, you are embarking on the journey of developing your academic research career.

This chapter will discuss steps to consider as you begin developing your research career. This is by no means an exhaustive list. But, it does represent tips we have learned from numerous successful academic surgical researchers who have shared what they consider important for a research career and what they wish they had known years ago. The tips also capture views of those who were unable to be successful academically and what they wish someone had shared with them.

Before You Start

Vision

If you are clear enough to know what you want in an academic surgical career, you want to consider the vision of what that research career will look like. As you interview for a job, you need to "sell" that vision to your future employer. If you don't

F. M. Johnston, MD, MHS (✉)
Department of Surgery, The Johns Hopkins University School of Medicine,
Baltimore, MD, USA
e-mail: fjohnst4@jhmi.edu

E. R. Haut, MD, PhD, FACS
Division of Trauma Surgery and Critical Care, Department of Surgery,
Johns Hopkins University School of Medicine, Baltimore, MD, USA
e-mail: ehaut1@jhmi.edu

© Springer International Publishing AG, part of Springer Nature 2018
K. Yoon-Flannery et al. (eds.), *A Surgeon's Path*,
https://doi.org/10.1007/978-3-319-78846-3_46

know what you want, you may not be taken as seriously as other candidates. Consider this: you are an investment for any surgical program. Just as if you are going to a meeting with a venture capital firm, you want to be able to "sell" your idea. If you can't articulate your vision and plan, then the program may not want to take a risk and hire you. If you have ever watched an episode of "Shark Tank," you know to come prepared. Understanding what direction you want to go in will be crucial to creating your foundation and allow your future bosses to help create an atmosphere that will be conducive to your success. By no means do you need to have a fully written grant, but you should be able to give broad strokes of your ideas. Are you a basic or translational scientist? Or a health services researcher? What do you want to study? What do you need to be successful? Think hard about these questions and have your answers ready. Your preparation will help to ground your thoughts and give clarity to your future employer.

Negotiation and Contracts

You have impressed them and they offer you a contract. Congratulations. You are almost there. But the work of contract negotiations for research should begin before you ever get that first written contract. Consider starting on your first or second interview. Often when you return for a second interview, it is important that you begin to identify who and what are the resources that you need to be successful.

Work with your current mentors to have an overview of what these things may be. Consider the environment. Do your potential partners support the kind of work you want to do? Does the institution have a track record supporting your genre of research? Are there mentors and collaborators within the institution? Are there equipment and other human capital present and is it available for your use? Will they allow you to apply for a K-award? These are just some of the questions you should ponder.

When asked to come for a second interview, request meetings with potential mentors and collaborators. Prepare questions for these individuals and others to allow for understanding of what is or isn't present at the institution. This will show your seriousness and focus on your future. If you have done your homework, you can negotiate for the resources you need. This is likely the only time you will be able to ask for certain things. It is uncomfortable for some, but it is necessary. Get over it! Importantly, you must always remember if it is not in your contract, it doesn't exist.

Consider negotiating for protected research time. Ideally, 50% of your time would be protected to begin a hard-core research career. However, as you will find out, there are not many jobs offering this, so you have to consider what else you may be able to get. If you are offered 25% protected time but are placed in a very encouraging environment, this still may be the best option. You can ask for other resources (lab technician, database manager, research assistant, research nurse, and/or statistician). You may not get your own dedicated full-time employees, but even part-time staff to help start your work can be incredibly valuable. Other options to request include startup funding and/ or an agreement from a research mentor to share resources with you. Always look holistically at the job when you are negotiating your contract. Determine what they have and will they give you what you need to be successful. Never feel bad about asking for things, as long as you are reasonable.

Communication with Mentors and Collaborator

Before you start your first job interview and during the entire process, talk with your current mentors and collaborators. They will be invaluable sounding boards who can discuss potential pitfalls you may not see. They should also be able to give you insight into what to ask for during negotiations. As a mentee, don't be afraid to ask your mentor the hard questions. This is the pinnacle of the culmination of years of hard work. You want to get it right.

Ready to Begin!

You are about to begin your job. I hope you enjoyed your time off. Now it's time to get to work. The siren call of clinical volume will draw you to want to do more clinical work. While being the best clinician and surgeon you can be is important, remember your first year is crucial to set up your research and mentoring infrastructure to be productive. You likely have a ramp up in terms of how much clinical volume (cases, RVUs) is expected of you in the first year. Take advantage of this. If you are serious about being a true researcher, build your base and a strong foundation.

Meetings

When you begin, set up meetings to discuss in detail what the mentorship and collaborations will consist of going forward. There will be suggestions of other people to meet with who may provide other resources, ideas, and future collaborations. This takes time. Be thoughtful and come prepared. Prepare the other person for your meeting. Send them your CV, a paragraph about who you are and what you want to do, or even a specific aims page for a grant you are working on. Find out what you can about these individuals and their work and come with a list of questions and potential requests. You want to be focused, efficient, and effective with your time and theirs.

Teamwork

No matter what kind of research you will be doing, you are going to need a team. Meet with your team and outline your research goals and agenda. It is important that they are clear of your philosophy and priorities so they can help you accomplish them. While there will most certainly be a learning curve, it is important to set the tone for your team. Consider what you want to be their deliverables for each stage of your work. But always remember this is a team game and your success will be built off the ability of your team to be successful. Hire the best people and be organized in your work. This will pay dividends in the long run leading to successful attainment of more research funding.

Space

If possible, try to get dedicated "lab" space. This will be obvious for the basic scientists who need cell culture faculties or animal surgery suites. However, it is also important for the health services researchers too. You need somewhere to house your students, residents, post-docs, and other team members. If you are going to have primary research mentor, ask for an office (or at least a desk/cubicle) embedded within their lab. You will want a place to get away to do research, truly protected from clinical and the inevitable request from a partner to cover or your nurse to just see one quick patient.

Coordinate

An often-overlooked component of your research life that should be a main focus is coordination and scheduling of your time. Within the framework of your clinical responsibilities, consider how you work best and schedule your time to maximize your efficiency. If you are a "morning person," use that time to write. You only have so many hours in the day and you have to determine what to do with it. Being organized will help you to commit time and accomplish many of your goals. This is a time to be introspective, honest, and realistic with yourself.

Work closely with your assistant early on to block your schedule and protect time. This will be an iterative process that will require you to meet frequently as you get more accustomed to a work and home schedule. Embrace the process! Organize your days so you will be most productive, and plan in advance for experiments, writing, and meetings. Create a template to document when you will be submitting grants and work backward including time to submit to your institutional grants team. Consider blocking additional time in the weeks prior to grant submissions to allow time with little interruption or distraction. Ultimately, organization will put you in the mindset to be at your most productive.

Write

You are going to hear this a lot when you begin your research career. Write, write early, and write often. Writing is part of your job, just like clinic, rounds, and surgery. This is easier said than done and will require significant patience to accomplish. Consider why it is important to write and what you can do to overcome barriers to our success in writing. You want to produce good work. This is your output upon which you will be judged.

The most successful academic surgeons write every day. While this may seem impossible at first, you can learn to do this just as with any other skill. Start with smaller chunks of time. By titrating in some writing, over time you will be more productive. You will have a tough time finding a 4-h block to write. Use 15–30-min blocks instead. You will be amazed how much you can get done. Consider joining a "writing accountability group" or something similar if your institution offers one. The positive peer pressure from your colleagues will help immensely.

To be a successful researcher, grant funding should be a goal. If you want to write a grant, this is not a short-term process. This is something that you need to be working on for at least 6 months prior to your submission for larger proposals. You want to write the best proposal possible, so take the time to write a little each day and have enough time to send it to mentors and collaborators who will help to perfect your work. Grant reviewers all agree that an application with typos and grammatical errors turns them off to the rest of the proposal. Even if you have great science, your proposal may be dead on arrival. Grantsmanship is a skill that needs to be honed just as any research or clinical skill. Consider attending a grant-writing workshop sponsored by your university or a national organization (i.e., the Association for Academic Surgery/Society of University Surgeons). This will ultimately pay long-term dividends if done early and right.

Mentoring

Mentoring is an important and honored component of our jobs. This responsibility should not be taken likely. Before you agree to be a research mentor, consider the following. Understand what it is to be a mentor and what your role will be. There are many articles, websites, and blogs that highlight the role of the mentor and mentee. Take time to consider the points that are raised. This is by no means a static relationship and you will grow in your role. However, your time and effort is crucial so please consider doing your homework so that you and your mentee can be most efficient and effective. Before you meet with a potential research mentee, consider what you will ask of them. Ask yourself the tough questions. Do I have the resources for them to be productive? Do I have the time to work closely with them? How much effort will they need from me? While mentees will come with many different skill levels, take note of what their skills and experiences are and determine does their skill level match with what I would like them to do? Don't offer to mentor or ask for a mentee until you are ready. If the mentee is not successful, that is as much a reflection on you as them. Fair or not this is the reality so be thoughtful and have a regimented plan of action. Be structured in what you ask from them and stick to its concrete output. Know yourself and work within those parameters for a successful relationship.

Support

This last section asks you to consider some logistical components of your research life. Understanding, addressing, and embracing these components will lead to a more fruitful research career and easier life in the long run.

Financial

Research costs money and someone needs to pay for it. You (hopefully) have some funding either in the form of startup funds provided by your department, extramural grant funding, or philanthropy. You need to manage this money. You are responsible for keeping track of these funds and have responsibility for how they are allocated. In some instances, other people may be relying on you (e.g., research technician or research assistant). You should meet with financial manager of your department and clearly identify who your point person is to contact in regard to how your money is allocated and tracked. Ask for a tutorial regarding how they budget the components of their spreadsheet. Try to meet with these individuals on a regular basis at first until you have a full grasp of how your money is being spent.

Grant Submissions

If you will be submitting grants, learn the landscape for grant submission within your institution. Plan to be well ahead of the timeline you are told. Be prepared for issues that may arise that are outside of your control. Many federal grants have just a few common deadlines and you will likely be submitting around the same time as the seasoned researchers. These larger grants may take up more time from grant and budget specialist in your institution. Prevent the heartburn that may come with a message that requires your expeditious response in the last few days before final submission. Often this may require you to need things from others who may not have the time you do. Get letters of recommendation and bio sketches as early as possible. These small pieces can make or break you. Understanding and controlling your local circumstances as much as possible will go a long way to your early and continued success.

Personal

Soon, you have more control over your schedule than you ever have before. While this is somewhat freeing you now also have more responsibilities than you probably ever had before. Take time to spend with your significant other. Make sure to consider your personal and familial responsibilities. If you have children, obtain dates for events in advance and schedule your time around this. Schedule time for the gym, or a run, or a tennis match, or whatever else is important outside of work. With multiple diverse demands on your time, there will most certainly be some trial and error but you can do this.

Closing

Good luck as you begin your research career. The journey will likely have great highs and lows. It will frustrate you at times, but if you are thoughtful and use the resources available, you will find it a fulfilling career choice. Always remember you are not alone. As you embark, share your tales and experiences with your colleagues. Learn from each other. Often, peer mentorship is even better than senior guidance.

Chapter 47
Continuing Medical Education/ Maintenance of Certification

Carla Fisher

So you passed your boards? Congrats! While this is one of the most important steps in your post-residency or fellowship career, you need to stay vigilant about tracking your continuing medical education (CME) soon after you pass your boards (or at least soon after you start your first job). The concept of "Maintenance of Certification" or MOC is an admirable and reasonable one. It represents a surgeon's ongoing commitment to professionalism, lifelong learning, and practice improvement following initial certification. The best overall resource for this topic is to go right to the source (www.absurgery.org/default.jsp?exam-moc). The goal of this chapter is to give an overview of what this means and provide some pointers as this can seem daunting, especially while building and maintaining a busy practice. The best advice I can give is to pay attention to this early so that you are not scrambling to meet the requirements right before they are due.

There are four components of the MOC. The initial step is relatively simple and involves the acquisition of your medical license, establishing and sharing your hospital credentials, and obtaining letters of references from the chief of surgery and/or chair of credentials at your institution. The website mentioned above overviews this, and you will receive correspondence to prompt you to do this.

Part 2, or lifelong learning and self-assessment, is the one *you want to pay attention to* when you are starting in practice. I can't emphasize enough that documentation is essential for this portion of MOC. Essentially this requires keeping track of any Category 1 CME credits relevant to your practice over a 3-year cycle. You have just completed 5–7 years of CME, so that's great, but now you need to document that you are going to continue to be a lifelong learner, and as you know, if it is not documented somewhere, it didn't happen! At most hospitals you can receive CME

C. Fisher, MD
Department of Surgery, Indiana University School of Medicine,
Indianapolis, IN, USA
e-mail: fishercs@iu.edu

© Springer International Publishing AG, part of Springer Nature 2018
K. Yoon-Flannery et al. (eds.), *A Surgeon's Path*,
https://doi.org/10.1007/978-3-319-78846-3_47

235

credits for attendance at *grand rounds, morbidity and mortality conference*, and potentially other educational lectures or events such as journal club. As a side note, there are strict requirements for establishing a lecture or event that grants people CME credits and may be something you want to look into if you set up a recurring event (such as a journal club) at your institution. *At many institutions, these are recorded electronically, and at the end of the year, or anytime, you will be able to access this site and capture all of the CME credits you have earned.* If this is not the case, then it is essential that you track these hours yourself. The hours will still have to be tracked by your institution, but they may be harder to find when you need them. When onboarding at your new job, ask about this and give yourself a reminder to access this website or information once/year to keep for your records.

Another option for obtaining CME credits is to attend regional or national conferences. These meetings can be fun and a great way to catch up with colleagues, but obviously the most important part of a meeting is the education, so make sure you get credit for this! This could be a national meeting (American College of Surgeons), or it could be a local or regional meeting. Either way this is usually a way to really supplement your learning and earn a lot of CME credits. Time at conferences can take you away from your job for several days at a time. For people in academics, this might be expected of you and easier to navigate. If you are in a private practice, you are still expected to maintain your MOC, but leaving for these meetings may be harder to integrate in your practice. As part of your negotiation (best scenario) or after you are hired, you should find out how much financial support you receive for these conferences and if there is dedicated time set aside to attend. Keep in mind that MOC is an *expected* part of your job, and your employer should support this financially and otherwise. For most meetings, you are expected to fill out evaluations and sometimes take tests to receive your credits. I would recommend making a note as soon as you finish a meeting to go online (or whatever they ask you to do) to obtain this credit. Usually you will receive a certificate with the amount of credits you have received. I have a folder at my desk where I put these certificates, which is essential for easy accessibility.

For the American Board of Surgery, they currently require 90 Category 1 credits every 3 years. Perhaps more importantly, 60 of these credits must include self-assessment that essentially means that you were "quizzed" on the content of the lecture. You must obtain 75% correct, and there is no limit to how many times you can take a self-assessment test. When you become board certified, your board certification test will count as these 60 self-assessment credits, so you are off the hook for this requirement for the first 3-year cycle!

The key to maintaining MOC, and not creating an unnecessary headache for yourself, is documentation and recordkeeping of any CME-eligible activities you participate in.

The third component of MOC involves your recertification exam. The final component is ongoing participation in a local, regional, or national outcome registry or quality assessment program and will be discussed in the next section.

Tracking Cases (and Other Stuff)

It is very important that you have some method to track your surgical cases and, in some case, patients that you see in the clinic. There are many different ways, and reasons, to do this.

It is absolutely essential to start keeping track of your cases when you begin your first job. For practical purposes, you will need the procedures you have performed over a year to become a fellow of the American College of Surgeons. Also, if you transfer jobs, it is possible that they will want to see a list of procedures you have performed over the previous few years. It is also essential that you keep track of your cases for billing purposes. Whether you are in private practice (more important) or academics (still important), there will likely be coders who are submitting your cases, but it is important to cross-check these submissions with your own data. You may receive paperwork from your employer indicating that you performed and billed for six cholecystectomies in a given month, but you have ten cases listed. This can absolutely happen, but you will never know if you are not tracking your cases. This can be especially easy to do and set up as a routine when you start in practice and are not as busy.

The next question is how you want to track these cases. For my first job, I opened a (secure) excel spreadsheet and just started tracking information (name, date of birth, diagnosis, procedure). I think, at the very least, this is what you need. As a resident I kept stickers in a book and then added them to the case log system. I do not think that "stickers" are the best way for keeping track of cases as an attending, and likely these will be a thing of the past at some point in the future. For some of the reasons mentioned above, you need something that can be easily submitted online or sent via email. Along those lines, *it is essential* that your documentation is HIPAA compliant. This could be a secure document, use of de-identified patient information or some other methods to ensure that you are compliant. In addition to basic information about the case, it is important for surgeons to know their reoperative rate or complication rate, etc., and this provides a method to have this information for yourself in real time.

In addition to surgical cases, you should consider what additional information might be helpful to track as you move forward in your practice. As surgeons, we understand the importance of tracking surgical cases, but should you also be tracking information related to office visits? How many new patients did you see last month, and how does that compare to the prior year or your partner? Your institution is likely tracking this information for you but, it is always helpful to be able to compare the institutional data to your own.

Besides individual tracking of cases (and other stuff), your institution may be tracking this information in the form of a local database, and there are also national databases through various surgical societies that you can enter into as well. I am referring back to *part 4 of your MOC* as well. The American College of Surgeons has recently launched the Surgeon Specific Registry (SSR). The goal of these large registries is to track cases and outcomes in a convenient, easy-to-use way, and many allow you to log via your computer or mobile device. They fulfill part of your MOC (bonus!) and allow easy transmittal of cases to the American Board of Surgery for recertification. Breast surgeons have the option of entering their cases in the Mastery of Surgery program through the American Society of Breast Surgeons. This is a nice way to add to a growing database and allow for meaningful information on both a small (individual) and large basis. For instance, you can pull your own reports for re-excision rates and stages of cancer, and you don't have to calculate this on your own. Programs like this can also help keep surgeons on track and provide helpful notifications when you may not have staged a patient appropriately. This type of information can be especially important for the early surgeon or the surgeon in a smaller or private practice. One of the "disadvantages" of these types of registries is the time required to enter all of the information. While the yield is higher, it is the difference between a few seconds to enter patient information in an excel spreadsheet and potentially 5–15 min to enter individual patients in a larger, more comprehensive registry. I will refer you back to the website at the beginning of the chapter for more information about these registries. There are many acceptable programs for part 4 of MOC, and if you are at a large academic center, you will certainly meet this requirement with your institutional tracking.

Happy tracking!

Chapter 48
Board Exams

Marc Neff

Board exams are a necessary evil to the practice of medicine in the twenty-first century. They are the last hurdle in a long line of tests that included exams to get into medical school, exams to get your license, and in-service exams through residency. Depending on your specialty, there may be some unique differences in what it takes to become board certified. I will focus here on the General Surgery Board Exam.

The written part, otherwise referred to as a qualifying exam, is just another exam like any other you have taken. Many of the questions will test your knowledge and test your ability to read questions properly. The exams also test your endurance and your ability to keep your focus through the 8-hour exam. The following is taken from the American Board of Surgery (ABS) website:

- The General Surgery Qualifying Examination (QE) is offered annually as the first of two exams required for board certification in general surgery. The exam consists of about 300 multiple-choice questions designed to evaluate a surgeon's knowledge of general surgical principles and applied science.
- It is a 1-day exam lasting approximately 8 h and is held at computer-testing facilities across the USA. The exam is administered in five 90-min sessions, with optional 10-min breaks between sessions, and one longer 40-min break offered between the third and fourth session. Once a session has concluded, you will not be able to revisit those questions.
- Results are posted approximately 4 weeks after the exam; you will be notified by an email when they are available.

The exam's content outline is available as a pdf for download. Individuals who complete general surgery residency will have no more than 7 academic years immediately following residency to become certified. There is also a requirement to submit an operative experience report that is deemed acceptable to the ABS, not only as to volume but also as to spectrum and complexity of cases.

M. Neff, MD, FACS, FASMBS
Center for Surgical Weight Loss, Jefferson Health New Jersey, Cherry Hill, NJ, USA

© Springer International Publishing AG, part of Springer Nature 2018
K. Yoon-Flannery et al. (eds.), *A Surgeon's Path*,
https://doi.org/10.1007/978-3-319-78846-3_48

The scarier part for most applicants is the oral exam, also known as the certifying exam, again taken from the American Board of Surgery (ABS) website:

- The General Surgery Certifying Examination (CE) is the last step toward board certification in general surgery. It is an oral exam consisting of three consecutive 30-min sessions, each conducted by a team of two examiners.
- The CE's purpose is to evaluate a candidate's clinical skills in organizing the diagnostic evaluation of common surgical problems and determining appropriate therapy. Emphasis is placed on candidates' ability to use their knowledge and training to safely, effectively, and promptly manage a broad range of clinical problems.
- The CE is held five times per academic year in major US cities. CE dates and sites for the next academic year are posted on this website in late spring. Once CE sites are posted, eligible candidates should select a site as soon as possible and must select a site by Sept. 1. Failure to select a site is considered a lost opportunity.
- All candidates are offered no more than one opportunity per academic year in each year of admissibility to take the CE. If you fail to select a CE site, or opt not to take the CE in a given year, it is a lost opportunity.

Yes, this all sounds very scary, but it's just the administrative stuff that goes with anything like this. The important part in the information above is that the exam tests the candidate's ability to be a sound and safe general surgeon. The oral exam is the last mountain to climb for the surgical trainee. Often mentioned at M&M conferences for the past 5 years as "what is the board answer" or "you will fail if you say that on your boards." Enough buildup has been made of the exam to strike fear into the hearts of any surgical attending. It's an amazing memory I have of sitting in the prep room with attending surgeons and recent fellowship graduates and looking around the room to see everyone pale and diaphoretic, with quivering hands shifting in their seats, waiting for the exam to begin. I didn't notice that the first time around as I was one of them, but the second time, after a good meal, a drink, and a good night sleep, confident in my knowledge and ability to answer safely, I did.

There are courses to take to prepare one for the oral exam. I, sadly, had an opportunity to take one of these courses twice. I highly recommend them. The exam is more about your confidence and your ability to take hours/days/weeks of real-life clinical workup and postoperative care and boil it down to 10 min of high yield facts, thoughtful safe decision making, and nothing that sounds experimental or shooting from the hip. The examiners are supposed to get you outside of your comfort zone, give you the curve balls, and make you think on your feet. Don't be a cowboy/cowgirl. Give the safe answer. Don't expect to describe the latest greatest technique that you just read about in the *Journal of Irreproducible Results* and expect to pass or impress the examiners. They don't want to be impressed with your knowledge. You can't impress them with your skill. Their job is to determine if you will be a safe surgeon with the seal of the American Board of Surgery behind you. Trust what you have been taught and don't overthink it.

Chapter 49
Becoming a Fellow of the American College of Surgeons and American College of Osteopathic Surgeons

Asanthi M. Ratnasekera and Marc Neff

Introduction

So you have passed your boards, and you are settling into your new attending life. The next step is to become a fellow of the American College of Surgeons (ACS) or American College of Osteopathic Surgeons (ACOS). In order to become a fellow, there are several criteria that need to be met.

ACS Requirements

The ACS encourages the application for fellowship to assess your practice and to ensure that your practice is according to the standards of the college. There are some requirements that must be met. For detailed listings of the criteria, please refer to the website at https://www.facs.org/member-services/join/fellows/fellowreq.

- You must have graduated from a medical school acceptable to the American College of Surgeons.
- You must have a certification of specialty practice by an American Surgical Specialty Board or an American Osteopathic Surgical Specialty Board or an appropriate specialty certification by the Royal College of Physicians and Surgeons of Canada.
- You must have a full and unrestricted license to practice medicine and have no action pending against you.

A. M. Ratnasekera, DO (✉)
Crozer-Keystone Health System, Upland, PA, USA

M. Neff, MD, FACS, FASMBS
Center for Surgical Weight Loss, Jefferson Health New Jersey, Cherry Hill, NJ, USA

© Springer International Publishing AG, part of Springer Nature 2018   241
K. Yoon-Flannery et al. (eds.), *A Surgeon's Path*,
https://doi.org/10.1007/978-3-319-78846-3_49

- You must have 1 year of surgical practice after the completion of all formal training.
- Have a current appointment on the surgical staff of the applicant's primary hospital.
- Have a current surgical practice that establishes the applicant as a specialist in surgery.
- Have professional proficiency as determined by the fellows you have listed as references.
- Have interest in pursuing professional excellence both as an individual surgeon and a member of the surgical community.

Once the criteria are met, an online application must be filled out along with a fee. You must ask current fellows to act as your references. You must also submit a list of cases from the 12 months after formal training is completed.

Once the application is received and reviewed, the board may make one of three decisions: approval, postponed, or denial. The postpone decision may be given to allow the applicant to acquire more experience. Denial applications may be appealed and reversed. However, following a denial application, the applicant must wait a 3-year period prior to reapplying.

If your application is approved, congratulations! You will be admitted into the fellowship during the Ceremony at the Clinical Congress each year in October.

ACOS Requirements

The ACOS has similar requirements to ACS. The ACOS has criteria that must be met based on three categories. You must have certain amount of points accumulated between the three categories. The three categories are National AOA and ACOS appointments, Educational, and State and Local contributions and appointments. The criteria that are included in the first category are the ACOS and AOA conferences you have attended, Surgical Board certification, and ACOS membership. The educational category requires you to list any lectures you have done, any journals or articles published, or any presentations at state or national conferences. The state and local contributions category requires you to list any local, hospital, state, or national committee membership you hold. Each of these activities is assigned points. Please refer to the ACOS website for detailed listings available at http://www.facos. org/OS/Membership/Fellowship_Application/OS/Navigation/Membership/ FACOS_Designation.aspx.

Once you have achieved all the required points, you are to fill out an application, along with a fee. Two letters of recommendation from current fellows of the ACOS is required. The decisions are similar to ACS application. If you are approved, you must assign a fellow to "hood" you during the college's ceremonial conclave the same year of application.

Part V
Long-term Goals and Planning

Chapter 50
Learning New Procedures

Marc Neff

After I graduated from a surgical residency and a minimally invasive surgical fellowship (MIS), I figured I knew all I needed to know. Even my fellowship director tried to temper my brash declaration that I knew all the MIS had to offer by reminding me that medicine changes and that I was likely only to be about 10 years ahead of everyone else. He couldn't have been more correct. I graduated fellowship in 2003. By 2005, I was attending my first course on sleeve gastrectomies. I attended one more course and reviewed the world's literature at the time and did my first sleeve in 2007. The lessons from that time are included in this chapter.

There is a level of safety in experimenting and learning in surgical residency and fellowship that doesn't exist after graduation. While training, you are expected to make mistakes, you anticipate being taught, and you listen, sometimes begrudgingly, to the advice of your instructors and mentors because they know more than you do and have more experience. All of that disappears after training is complete. If you attempt to learn a new procedure, it is all on you. It can affect your referrals, your reputation, put you at risk for serious battles in your department, and even affect our malpractice. Sadly, and I say with almost 100% certainty, at some point in your career, you will be learning a new technique, device, or procedure.

Performing my first sleeve gastrectomy was quite daunting. First, there was reviewing the current state of the literature, finding a course, traveling to it, taking lots of notes, talking to the instructors during and afterward, and getting real data on real patients. I even went to a second course from a different industry sponsor with different instructors to be sure I wasn't missing anything. Then I had to find a patient who was prepared to be the first case and give them the appropriate disclaimers. Getting the appropriate mentor to come to my institution and getting them credentialed and paid was yet another hurdle in a seemingly unending number of hurdles. I had to convince my partner it was an appropriate surgery to pursue and figure out how to get the insurance companies to pay for the procedure. I trained all the staff

M. Neff, MD, FACS, FASMBS
Center for Surgical Weight Loss, Jefferson Health New Jersey, Cherry Hill, NJ, USA

© Springer International Publishing AG, part of Springer Nature 2018
K. Yoon-Flannery et al. (eds.), *A Surgeon's Path*,
https://doi.org/10.1007/978-3-319-78846-3_50

in the office, OR, dieticians, and nurses on the floor what to expect and how to interact with the patient. There were many times I wanted to quit. Convincing your institution's department chair and credentialing office to do something "experimental" is quite a challenge. And, after even a couple of years of doing the procedure, I then had to face someone joining our staff who claimed to have more experience, better outcomes, and told me much of what I was doing was completely wrong. A hard lesson learned in humility, patience, and propaganda. In the end, after many gray hairs, there was a happy ending. I am now the first in my region who performed a laparoscopic sleeve gastrectomy and that has done wonders for my reputation and growth of my practice.

So, if you decide you want to be the first, take a step back and take out a piece of paper and make some real plans. You have to get trained and get all the appropriate certificates. You have to have a preceptor prepared to come to your institution to monitor your first cases. You have to train all of your staff. You have to speak with everyone that patient will interact with from your billing staff, to your front desk staff, to the answering service. You need to think out every contingency plan and strategize every possible outcome. You need to have frank discussions with your hospital, department, partners, and the patient. You may even need to create a separate surgical consent form just for the procedure. You also need to be prepared for failures, or rather "disguised learning opportunities," along the way. A discussion with your malpractice carrier wouldn't hurt. If you haven't figured it out yet, this is going to take *a lot* of time, time away from seeing office patients and time away from the OR and time to train in a lab and time away from your family. Time is one of our most valuable possessions, and as you have so little free time as an attending surgeon, be sure that the time invested in learning a new procedure is going to have an appropriate return on investment.

Lastly, I strongly suggest that you collect your own data and stay current with the literature. Put on your surgical scientist hat and subject yourself to the same scrutiny you would give to a journal article, even its references.

Chapter 51
Robotic Surgery

Matias J. Nauts and Roy L. Sandau

The use of robotics in surgery in general has been an established idea and in certain specialties is considered the standard of care. In general surgery, however, robotics is still in its adolescence but has been exponentially gaining ground and popularity. Today laparoscopic and traditional open procedures outnumber robotic-assisted general surgery procedures. The technology has improved, and pioneering surgeons have pushed the limits of what is possible on the robotic platform. The world of robotic surgery has changed vastly over the last 10 years; there has been a surge of general surgeons taking to the console. For the majority of these general surgeons, training on the da Vinci surgical system was done after their formal training found during traditional internship, a general surgery residency, and fellowship. These practicing surgeons have taken the leap of faith to learn a new and cutting edge technique, and now formal robotic training is offered in many of the general surgery residency programs and advanced minimally invasive fellowships.

There currently are two paths that a general surgeon can take to become certified and adequately trained to perform robotic surgeries. The first is the one taken by the resident or fellow who are fortunate enough to be in a training program that offers robotic surgical experience. The second path, and the most common, is taken by the currently practicing general surgeon who learns outside of residency on how to use the robot. Each of these routes is equally as difficult in a different way, takes time and commitment to master, but is well worth the investment.

The training offered to residents and fellows begins as observation, where the trainee will observe a skilled robotic surgeon during a case and learn about the different components of the robotic system. The trainee will also be expected to

M. J. Nauts, DO (✉)
Laparoscopic and Robotic General Surgery, Christus Surgical Group Lake Charles,
Lake Charles, LA, USA

R. L. Sandau, DO, FACOS
Department of Surgery, Jefferson Health New Jersey, Cherry Hill, NJ, USA

© Springer International Publishing AG, part of Springer Nature 2018   247
K. Yoon-Flannery et al. (eds.), *A Surgeon's Path*,
https://doi.org/10.1007/978-3-319-78846-3_51

complete online da Vinci-provided modules that will further teach them about how to use the robotic system. After the completion of the modules, the trainee will be allowed to assist at bedside, learn how to dock the arms, load instruments, and then finally sit on the console. The amount of time in cases the resident or fellow is allowed to perform varies among teaching institutions; therefore not all general surgeons graduating today will be proficient in robotic surgery. Eventually the training resident will be focused more on working on the console, increasing surgical proficiency, and learning new techniques and procedures on the robotic platform. A graduating resident who is proficient with robotic surgery should be able to identify patients appropriate for the robotic approach, aid the robotic team during the setup of cases, and complete procedures efficiently on the console with minimal conversion rates.

For surgeons who are not fortunate enough to receive robotic training during residency or fellowship training, there is a structured program offered by da Vinci to teach general surgeons the tools needed to operate on their robotic system. The program is structured to provide basic understanding of the technology and relies on both self-directed practice and on-site training. The da Vinci training program includes multiple phases which build up on each other to teach new robotic surgeons safe principles to ensure success. The first step before embarking on robotic training is to contact your local da Vinci representative as they will be your greatest asset during the training phase and early implementation phase.

Phase 1 starts with a basic overview of the da Vinci robotic system. During this phase the budding robotic surgeon will be introduced to all the parts of the surgical system and be allowed to sit and work on the console in simulated exercises. The surgeon will also be taken to other hospitals that have been set up as observation sites. Here the surgeon will see live cases and interact with established robotic surgeons who are experts in all robotic technologies and applications.

Phase 2 gets into more detail and specifics regarding the technology. The surgeon is given online modules that have been created on how the system works, common pitfalls, optimizing port placement, and the basic knowledge to use the system efficiently. Simulations and drills will be performed on what is called a "dry box." This allows the robot to be docked, and the surgeon can sit at the console and perform skills that mimic maneuvers used during real surgery. Examples of some of the skills are intracorporeal suturing, maneuvering the camera, and passing things from one instrument to another, just to name a few. Once these skills have been performed adequately, live tissue exercises at a da Vinci training center will be scheduled. Basic procedures such as cholecystectomies and colon resections will be performed on a porcine model to further enrich the instruction before moving onto an actual patient. Once all of these training steps have been successfully completed, the surgeon may proceed with surgery on a patient of their choice. Each hospital has different criteria for credentialing new robotic surgeons. An experienced robotic surgeon usually has to proctor the initial cases, and the number of proctored cases is institution dependent.

There may be various barriers encountered on the road to becoming a proficient robotic surgeon. These barriers range from administrative resistance, financial, time constraints, availability of the robot, properly trained robotic staff, anxiety over learning something new, fear of poor outcomes, introducing new technology in the OR, and the list goes on. Many surgeons develop an interest for robotic surgery, but unfortunately can find the learning curve to be steep and frustrating. However, it can ultimately be a rewarding experience.

It is important to remember the robotic surgery is another surgical instrument, another tool in your surgical bag. When you start your training, do not think of the robot as something new or foreign. You already know how to complete the planned procedure. When surgeons first began laparoscopic surgery, they had to learn how to use new instruments and techniques to complete the surgery in similar fashion to the open approach. Robotic surgery combines the best of both approaches. The better 3D visualization and wristed instruments allow for minimally invasive surgery with open dexterity of movement. Sure there are gifted laparoscopic surgeons who can complete the same procedures, but robotic surgery enables the surgeons who have difficulty to transition to more advanced laparoscopic surgeries, beyond appendectomies and cholecystectomies to complex hernias, colon resections, paraesophageal hernias, and anything imaginable.

We had to prove to the administration in two different hospital systems that robotic general surgery was faster, safer, and profitable. We had to do our own research on outcomes and compare our data between laparoscopically and open. We had to show our results against the rest of the laparoscopic and open surgeons in the region. In the end, both hospitals eventually granted advanced robotic privileges in general surgery. What we found was that the learning curve for robotic surgery was around 20 cases for colorectal surgery and 15 cases for hernias. Our length of stay was reduced by a one full day for colorectal surgery compared to laparoscopic. Our cost for robotic hernia was cheaper than laparoscopic, and length of stay was short for both open and laparoscopic.

You really have to be "all in" to be proficient in robotics and cannot just dabble in it. But that goes with anything in surgical competencies, everything we do in the OR as surgeons is muscle memory and repetition. High-volume surgeons have always shown to have short operative times, better outcomes, and less complications. At this point every patient that walks in is a candidate for robotic approach. Revision surgery is generally easier on the robot. In our opinion, the best tool for lysis of adhesions is the da Vinci robotic platform. The operative times can also increase the more experience you have due to resident involvement and training.

It is also paramount to have good mentors and support. You may not be so lucky to have a local expert that you can call or text. Fortunately, we do have social media where you can have access to thousands of surgeon in all specialties to offer support and opinions about cases. Some Facebook groups that we belong to and have found resourceful include the Robotic Surgery Collaboration, International Hernia Collaboration, and SAGES Foregut Surgery Master's Program Collaboration. Using these resources may also help bolster your robotics training experience.

Chapter 52
Military Surgery

Gustavo Lopes

The economic pressure that today's young physicians face is tremendous. The average debt of graduating medical students continues to rise each year, creating significant long-term financial challenges. New doctors essentially have the equivalence of a mortgage payment without a house to show for it. For those who are debt adverse and willing to serve their country, the military offers an opportunity to pay for medical education through service.

The majority of military physicians enter the armed services through a scholarship program called the Health Professions Scholarship Program (HPSP). The program is offered by the Air Force, Army, and Navy. The Marine Corps' physicians are supplied by the Navy. Each service runs its program independently with slight variations.

Typically, candidates will apply for the scholarship prior to starting medical school or during medical school. Acceptance into medical school is a prerequisite to getting offered a scholarship, although the application process can start prior. The application process includes an interview, physical examination, and meeting eligibility requirements to join the military. Scholarships range from 1 to 4 years. For each year of scholarship, the student incurs 1 year commitment or "payback" to be served on active duty after the completion of residency. Residency time, even if served in active duty, does not count toward the students' obligation.

The scholarship covers all of the tuition costs, fees, books, and supplies for medical school. In addition, there is a monthly stipend paid to help with living expenses. Depending on the current recruitment needs, there may also be a potential sign-on bonus.

Once accepted into the program, students are commissioned as officers to the rank of second lieutenant in the Air Force and Army and Ensign in the Navy. During

G. Lopes, DO
General, Laparoscopic, and Robotic Surgery, Chairman Department of Surgery,
Martin Health Systems, Stuart, FL, USA

medical school, students are in the inactive reserves. However, there is a 45-day Active Duty Tour (ADT) requirement per year. This obligation can be met a number of ways and is not burdensome. Typically, the first year's ADT is completed with officer training between first and second year of medical school. Think of this as "basic training" specifically designed for doctors and dentists. The second, third, and fourth ADTs are typically completed as elective clinically rotations as part of third and fourth years of medical school. The students can schedule the rotations in the specialty of their choice at a military teaching hospital. Students are paid active duty rates during ADTs. Outside of ADTs, there are no other commitments during medical school.

Students are automatically promoted to the rank of Captain (Air Force and Army) or Lieutenant (Navy) at graduation. The path at this point can vary. New military physicians will, at a minimum, complete an internship. This can be performed in a military or civilian hospital based on the "match" results. The military does have its own match for graduating HPSP students, which precedes the civilian match. After internship, physicians can become a General Medical Officer (GMO) or Flight Surgeon and fulfill their active duty obligation. Alternatively, a student can complete a full residency upon medical school graduation and fulfill his or her active duty obligation thereafter. Fellowships are also allowable, but approval is subject to military needs and may incur more obligations.

Besides the more common HPSP program, there are other ways to join the military as a physician. For the Gung-ho military types, there is the Uniformed Services University. This is a military medical school. Students actually go to school while on active duty collecting active duty pay. They do incur more obligation, 7 years, and are typically required to complete a residency at a military hospital. For those who initially passed on the military and HPSP but still want some serious financial help, there is a program called the Financial Assistance Program (FAP). This is for those physicians already in residency. The FAP pays a large yearly bonus and monthly stipend, while the physician is a resident. For each year of benefits, there is 1 year of obligation plus an additional year. There are also a number of loan repayment programs offered. Finally, the Reserves are another way to serve as a military physician part-time and can be joined even after residency.

Life as a military surgeon is much like that of a civilian surgeon, most of the time. While dressed in uniform to go to work, the day to day is often the same, clinic days mixed with operating days. The makeup of your practice is largely in your control within the constraints of the resources available at a military hospital.

There are several significant benefits of working within the military system. The patient population is significantly younger, fitter, and healthier. The older patients you see (i.e., retired military and family) tend to have had access to health care most of their lives and are therefore also healthier on average. Performing surgery on fit, healthy bodies is actually quite a pleasure and not very commonplace in the civilian world today.

The volume of patients and caseload is considerably less in the average military hospital compared to civilian counterparts. Since all military personnel are also paid by salary, there is no pressure to produce or compete. Caseloads are commonly shared fairly equally. Reasonable caseloads and healthier patients lead to better results, greater job satisfaction, and less burnout.

The price for these benefits, of course, is the potential for deployments. Deployments not only include assignments in combat zones but also taskings in many other military locations around the world. They can last from several weeks to a year or more depending on the branch and assignment. The military has done a fair job in organizing a system of rotations in an attempt to make deployments more predictable and evenly distributed. Having said that, war is unpredictable and the war machine has many moving parts. The system doesn't always work perfectly, or as promised. In the end, a military surgeon is still a military officer in an organization where the mission's needs come first. Therefore, the military surgeon must accept this fact and be flexible enough to adapt as needed. This does create its own stress and is often the point in which some decide not to join the military or not to stay in the military.

Although most military physicians leave the military once their commitment is up, many find life in the military fulfilling and choose to stay longer. There is a certain level of fulfillment that can only be achieved by participating in a cause greater than yourself. Most physicians understand this. The reward of serving your country is powerful and compels many to make a career in the military.

Chapter 53
Five-Year and Ten-Year Plans

Marc Neff

I never had a 5-year plan after residency was completed. I certainly never considered the idea of a 10-year plan. Looking back on the first 10 years after residency was completed, that was so—incredibly—foolish. I have accomplished so many of the goals I had set out to do when I was a young surgical intern, but I got lost many times along the way, and it cost me more time, money, and effort than it needed to. There is an inherent value to writing things down. There is a real value to planning what you want and when you want to achieve it by and how to get there. There is a value to sharing your goals and dreams with your partner. There is a value to assessing your position in your practice, hospital, and department each year to see if you are reaching your goals.

An example of this I learned from a local plastic surgeon who came to an area densely populated by plastic surgeons and wanted to plant roots. He started at the very bottom rung of the ladder but had a plan. He took all the ER call at all the local ERs. A job no established plastic surgeon wanted, to come in in the middle of the night to sew up some young kid's face, and dealing with shredded tendon from a snow blower paid pretty well. But the goal there was to start to build your reputation, get your name out there among doctors and patients, and start building your practice. He worked out of his father's office so overhead was low, slowly all the while building his cosmetic practice. He and his family lived in a town house and kept costs low. Soon he was taking consults for all the complicated wounds in the hospital that no busy plastic surgeon wanted to spend their time on, again building his reputation, making his name known, keeping his costs low, and building his cosmetic practice. Then he completed a hyperbaric oxygen course, and he was named the director of the wound care center. Nice stipend came with it, again building his reputation, making connections, keeping costs low, and building his cosmetic practice. Ten years later, he had his Bentley, his mansion, and his own office

M. Neff, MD, FACS, FASMBS
Center for Surgical Weight Loss, Jefferson Health New Jersey, Cherry Hill, NJ, USA

© Springer International Publishing AG, part of Springer Nature 2018   255
K. Yoon-Flannery et al. (eds.), *A Surgeon's Path*,
https://doi.org/10.1007/978-3-319-78846-3_53

with an attached surgery center, and he gave up the directorship, the wound care center, and most of the hospital consults and ER calls. His 10-year plan was ingenious. That's the example to follow.

After you finish training, there is an instant surge of relief—a sense of "it's my time now" and that everything should come easy and should come visit. Many young surgeons purchase a house and/or car that is too expensive, live larger than they can afford, and then are forever trying to deal with financial stress. Many young academic surgeons don't have a coherent plan for how they are going to work their way toward full professorship and meander around on projects and research that has little or very slow return on investment. Some surgeons rush to get married and have children right at the end of their training or after training is completed only to find a new layer of responsibility and stress that comes with a family. So what should a young surgeon do? Make a plan.

Just like the example of the young plastic surgeon who had a 5-year plan of building reputation, keeping office costs and family costs low, and saving capital for bigger purchases down the line, patience is a virtue. He could have purchased the office, the house, and the car early in his career, but what would it have gained him? The foundation wasn't there. The roots need time to dig deep. And later, the directorship and the wound care center and the eventual private office with an attached surgery center followed as the cosmetic practice was booming—all a matter of timing. Incidentally, the surgeon is still married with a family of three.

The point to this chapter is to take your team. Write down your wants and dreams. Sit with your accountant, lawyer, spouse, other family members, and mentors, and develop a coherent plan of how to get there. There are many ways to get up the mountain, and most surgeons get there, but a great many take a whole lot longer because they didn't stop to develop a plan, essentially, to build a map of the quickest way to the top.

Chapter 54
Changing Practices

David M. Schaffzin

There is no perfect job. Anyone telling you different is selling something. If you are looking to leave your current practice, your goal should be "better." Remember from training, what is the enemy of better? *Perfect*. When asked why I like my current position, I tell them that it is pleasant. Everyone who works here is pleasant—in my office, my hospital, and my endoscopy center. Pleasant is about as accurate a way to describe my job, my practice, my patients, my day…they are pleasant. I travel a little farther to get here, but I only get out of my car once (with rare exception). In the 7 years at my second practice, I am for the most part happy to drive to work, to drive home, to be in my office, to round at my hospital, and to operate/perform colonoscopy in these four places, all attached to one facility, where I do all of my procedures and all of my patients. Perfect…no, but I have never turned the car around and run for the hills.

Nearly 75% of physicians going into practice will switch jobs at least once. I actually knew early on in my career that I would not be spending my entire career in the group I had joined. I had gone to my group in my third year with them and asked if we could break off colorectal surgery and have a separate call. I was informed that the practice was not structured that way and was not planning on changing. Moreover, two of my colorectal partners actively practiced general surgery and enjoyed it. It was clear that long term, I would be moving on. Interestingly, my group also believed that I wouldn't be there long term following that conversation, so they hired another colorectal/general surgeon to replace me. There was no negative to this, he became busy, and there was plenty of volume for all. However, I had not given notice or even "officially" was looking to leave. In fact, it was nearly 3 more years until I did actually leave. I had learned to be patient and bide my time.

D. M. Schaffzin, MD, FACS, FASCRS
Clinical Assistant Professor of Surgery,
Drexel University College of Medicine, Philadelphia, PA, USA

St. Mary Medical Center, Center for Colon and Rectal Health, Inc., Langhorne, PA, USA

© Springer International Publishing AG, part of Springer Nature 2018   257
K. Yoon-Flannery et al. (eds.), *A Surgeon's Path*,
https://doi.org/10.1007/978-3-319-78846-3_54

When an interesting job was posted, I sent my CV with a cover letter. These days, it's all done electronically, but an actual letter stands out. Many groups called back, I interviewed with a few that would be a good fit. A local GI group had offices in both New Jersey and Pennsylvania, and I was seeing patients from across the river where there was already an established colorectal group. The group had a good reputation but did not offer many of my services. My "niche" wasn't even something I thought I would do in practice, but it's what was needed in a multispecialty group with other colorectal surgeons. I was trained in all aspects of colorectal surgery, and specialized in oncology, but I specifically was trained in pelvic floor disorders and the unique workup these patients needed.

Lesson 1: Make yourself a unique referral basis by offering something that no one else in your group does. It is something you can use to grow, and if needed to build a new practice elsewhere, and will define you in a field saturated by other similar physicians.

Private practice is about referrals and reputation. No one asks you where you trained except for your first job and the occasional patient that thinks you look too young to be a surgeon. Patients trust their doctors, and when another physician recommends you, they already have a positive opinion of you.

Lesson 2: Always call the referring doctor, thank them, and tell them what you found, that the patient did well, when would they like to see the patient again, etc. You are your own best PR firm. And in these days where most communications are electronic, a phone call is appreciated.

So I bided my time, and when the very same colorectal group who was losing patients to me from across the river was ironically looking to expand, I picked up the phone and called. After talking about what they do, what I do, and how we would likely build a complimentary practice with mutual growth, we arranged a meeting. Before that meeting, they called the very same referring doctors who used me in New Jersey and were informed of the good work I do for their patients, how I run an anal physiology lab which no one else regionally did, and how their patients were very happy with my care. By the time I met with the senior partner, the decision between me and two other doctors being considered was mostly made. These days, with Facebook, Twitter, Google, and the vast Internet as a whole, anyone can know a lot about you before ever meeting you. Within a week of that meeting, I was offered a job.

Lesson 3: Unless you are in urgent need to get out of your practice, you have time to get it all right the second time around. You know how to practice medicine, how to operate, how to bill, how to code, how to build a referral basis, and how to build a good reputation. Use those skills to negotiate a fair and equitable contract. Get a contract attorney, but you and the new practice can probably negotiate 95% of things up front. Once you have a contract, *then* you can give your notice to your current group.

Lesson 4: Have an exit strategy. Know what you are required to do to give notice. Do NOT give it prematurely; you may end up unemployed for a time (translation, no income). Do NOT leave before the allotted time in your contract, which could be construed as breach of contract, and lead to a legal battle, especially if there is bad blood. Know what your restrictive covenant is and what the laws in your state/region are—I know someone who had to go to court over the distance from their prior practice (20 miles) because it was not specified as "driving distance" vs. "radius from primary office." Don't give your prior practice ammunition to fight you on any grounds. It is worth neither the stress nor the legal fees.

Once I had my timeline figured out, I had to give 90-day notice. Get out your calendar, and figure it out to the day. For me, I was starting after a Christmas week vacation with family, so my last day was the day before we left, and my first day at my new practice was the Monday after we returned. Make sure your credentialing is complete and your licensure and DEA are up to date and in the appropriate state (I had to transfer my DEA to PA from NJ, even though the number doesn't change).

Lesson 5: Don't burn bridges. While there was a lot of speculation on if I would leave, it was a surprise when I actually gave notice. I kept it amicable; I worked hard right up to the day I left. I was a team player, never was bitter, said goodbye graciously, and left quietly. For the first few years, I kept my staff privileges at my prior institution. Nothing in my contract said I had to give them up, and as a safety net, I could have gone back in any capacity (employed, join another group, etc.) if the move had not worked out. It is far easier to stay on staff than to try to get back on staff anew. And again, play it by the book. Whatever was in your contract, unless truly unfair practices (hopefully you negotiated well the first time around), is the standard in most states. The moment you decide to leave, your only goal should be to move on without stress, without fighting, without animosity, and with your reputation intact.

Lesson 6: Transparency. Get a written guarantee that you get to review the books and finances. You may have to sign a nondisclosure agreement, but I know someone whose practice had fraudulently billed for procedures they did not actually do. Fraud is a federal offense punishable by fines, loss of license, loss of the ability to participate in Medicare, and possible jail time. Insist that you get to see the numbers of what you (and preferably the remaining physicians) bill, what each of your collections are, what insurance contracts you pay, what the staff makes, and what moneys are put into retirement. My first practice hid much from me, so I knew what I wanted to see up front this time. This turned out to be a really good thing, because I found hundreds of thousands of dollars worth of missed or incorrectly billed visits and surgeries. Very quickly, I became the financial officer and compliance officer, simply because I knew what to look for and what needed correcting. While you may not be invaluable, you will start benefitting the practice immediately. Showing this skill set up front at your interview is even better.

Lesson 7: Know exactly what you bill, how to code, what modifiers to use and when, what defines the different levels of new patient visits, new patient consults, established patient visits, Medicare inpatient consults vs. private insurer consults, and procedure codes. This is on-the-job training. Your first years in practice are all about how to operate, when not to operate, how to manage complications, and families and your home life. But all the while, learn everything you can on how to actually run a practice. You never know, you might even go out on your own.

Lesson 8: Knowledge is power. I recommend you use a program like SuperCoder or ACSCodingToday to see what is bundled together, what can be billed together, what a given procedure pays, how many RVUs it is worth, and when to use what modifier. If your practice doesn't use it, buy it yourself. No one knows better what you did in a surgery or office visit more than you. And the less the billing staff has to do to figure out about what you did, the faster they bill things out, and the sooner reimbursement comes in. Even in a hospital-based practice, you should know how many RVUs a given surgery has, and keep a record of everything you do so you have the information and power to go to others in a group and show them your worth (or worse, have to prove your worth in court). The American College of Surgeons has a Practice-Based Learning Website to save your case data in a HIPAA-compliant manner. It can run reports on case numbers, frequency, complications, and outcomes. It gives you the power to hand a report over showing exactly what your worth is, and whether this is your first practice or subsequent, you are your best cheerleader.

And so, a few phone conversations, a meeting, some lawyer stuff, and I left my multispecialty group to go back into private practice, now purely colorectal, with a better quality of life. I had to give up a few things (no separate death and dismemberment policy, for instance, and the IRA in my new practice was not one that matched a percentage of what was put away, and my wife's medical was the better of our two practices) to become what I had intended, a purely colorectal surgeon with some academic aspects. A nice bonus, we train residents from a local university hospital, so I'm more academic, and I joined a group with an excellent reputation, already established, where I could grow beyond the practice they had been for decades.

So this brings us back to the beginning of the chapter. You have decided to move on. Are you sure? How sure? How do you come to this decision? It may involve moving, selling your home, changing school systems, getting a license in a new state, taking a pay cut, or getting paid more but moving somewhere less metropolitan. True story: My wife (the urologist) was offered a job in Alexandria, *Louisiana*, circa 2006. The story goes that we were at a urologic drug meeting at Universal Studios in Florida (I was out on rides and introducing myself as Mister since it wasn't *my* Big Pharma conference, I got to be the tag along spouse and was loving it), back in the day when a drug company could fly you and a spouse down for a weekend, put you up at a hotel, take you to dinner, and even offer free park tickets. A urologist there made her an offer hard to refuse: 3 weeks of work per month PLUS 4 weeks of vacation a year, the worst payer was "225% of Medicare," and it was an HMO. And it was in Alexandria, *Louisiana*. A one-and-a-half hour drive from Houston (closest airport as parents were from Long Island, Pennsylvania, and California), with a new Wal-Mart, new Starbuck's, new 6-screen movie theaters, and low taxes and low cost of living. We would need to put the kids in private school, but on Realtor.com we could have 8 acres with a 6 BR 4½ bath home with a horse stable for the same as we could sell our 4-bedroom 0.5-acre house in New Jersey. My wife said she'd think about it and get back to them in a week. The urologist even picked up his cell and called the head of the regional multispecialty surgical group, who was happy to have me come down and talk. For me, it would have been a lateral move, still doing some general surgery, but similar quality of life for more pay. My wife asked a very insightful and important question, "Are there Jews there?" Turns out, just a few. I spoke with the local synagogue administrator (there was no rabbi). They rented a rabbinical student or cantor for the Jewish holidays, for the 200 families who came from a 100-mile radius, and the nearest Jewish Community Center (JCC) was a 4-h drive toward New Orleans. My reply, "We could do it, for like 5 years, and be debt-free." You can guess her response. And yes, we also know *that* doctor who tried and failed that plan. He thought that backwoods anywhere USA was doable for 5 years, and didn't make it 2, and his wife didn't make it one, but she left while he worked on getting out.

Lesson 9: So you are sure you want to leave your job. Make a list. Column A, what you dislike about your current practice. Column B, what you like about your current practice. Column C, what could be changed to make you stay. If needed, Column D, what the new job that it's worth turning your world around. Go over it again and again, talk it over with anyone who it would directly affect (spouse, significant other, and kids). Before you make the leap, decide if this is something you really NEED to do. Are you in a practice where you could take Column C to your current practice, rationally explain why you are considering leaving, and what they could do to alter that trajectory? There are times you *have* to leave, but there are times you may simply *want* to leave really badly. Starting over is not easy. But in the right situation, it may well be worth it. Be honest with yourself.

My former group was forced in my third year with them to become hospital employed. Now 10 years after that, they have left that healthcare system to go back into private practice. Of those in the group PRIOR to my joining (and not since retired), ALL have left to re-form the original private group, taking three additions from after me with them. For those who were junior to me or came after I left, all but two stayed with the hospital system. I left for different reasons, but clearly their plan had on some level failed. I am on good terms with all of them, and they keep me updated when I run into them at the gym or some gala. There is grass all around, some greener, some taller, some dying, some just in need of water, and some brown from too much water. I think I made the correct choice. It was not easy, and with healthcare changing annually, I always fear that we all will be forced to make similar choices in the future, maybe many times in a single career. More seasoned surgeons remember the "golden age of surgery," of high reimbursement and strong work ethics, where surgeons were respected simply for being a physician. Some brand-new surgeons haven't ever had to work more than 80 h in a week and will never know the days when only physicians (and drug dealers) carried beepers, and when one went off, a whole restaurant stopped eating dinner to watch the doctor go make a call, whispering "that's a doctor" and "I wonder if they have to go operate." Your best bet to have a great career is to find a place you will enjoy going to work, enjoy treating your patients, and enjoy being home with your family. Expectations, I tell patients, are as important as outcomes. Knowing as much as you can up front saves you a whole lot of issues after the fact. Once I finally understood many of the realities of practice, both private and hospital employed, I became much more realistic about what to expect and how to enjoy it. What you *wish* for may be very different from what you actually *want and need*. This is still a very noble profession and worthy of the time and sacrifice you put into it. If you start searching early, and are realistic about what you *want and need*, you will succeed.

Chapter 55
Leadership Development

Paula Ferrada

It is important to understand that leadership in medicine is a responsibility. Since very early on we influence others, first in our family environment or in our communities. Since surgical internship, our behavior influences everyone around us. Medical student recruitment can depend on how residents perceive their choice of career and, more importantly, how they voice their perceptions. Leading a team, having your voice heard, and advocating for the patient are examples of how we place our leadership skills to function in basic daily clinical activities.

There is a need for competent leaders in healthcare, who understand resource allocation, financial performance of an organization, and, most importantly, the well-being of patients we serve. Although some of the leadership traits are innate, the majority of tools that the leaders need to be efficient are learned. Power, although sometimes seen as an "evil" word, can have a positive connotation when referred to power over ourselves and our perception and that empowers others rather than powering through them.

Empowering others moreover empowers ourselves to be the best that we can be, to exert change when needed, and to stand together for fairness and transparency and is necessary in our professional environment. Understanding our power can lead to positive consequences and can help us see leadership not as a privilege but as a duty.

The sources of power in the civic arena are:

- Physical force: This is the power over others by means of violence. This kind of power is superficial and transitory. Dictatorships are an example of the use of physical force as means for power.

P. Ferrada, MD, FACS
Director of the Surgical Critical Care Fellowship, Surgical and Trauma ICU,
Virginia Commonwealth University, Richmond, VA, USA

Associate Professor of Surgery, Virginia Commonwealth University, Richmond, VA, USA
e-mail: Paula.ferrada@vcuhealth.org

© Springer International Publishing AG, part of Springer Nature 2018   263
K. Yoon-Flannery et al. (eds.), *A Surgeon's Path*,
https://doi.org/10.1007/978-3-319-78846-3_55

- Wealth: This refers of power by buying access to influence. It is also transitory.
- State action: This is the use of law to mandate behaviors in a community. Policies can be interpreted as frozen power since they perpetuate a particular flow of influence.
- Social norms: This is a softer source of power, however longer lasting. It refers to what the consensus of the community thinks is adequate behavior. These norms are difficult to change unless there is a shift in the needs of the community.
- Ideas and power in numbers: Ideas that motivate a critical number of individuals can be an endless source of power that can exert change even if other sources of power are present. Examples are the civil rights movement and gender equality.

Tools to Become a Good Leader

Finding Your Purpose

When we want to exert positive influence, it is important to understand the reasons why we are supporting an idea or changing a behavior. As a leader you must understand the reason why you want to seek change before sharing a strategy with the team you intent to lead. Finding the overlap between your mission, vision, profession, and vocation can be a good exercise to find your purpose (Fig. 55.1).

Once you know your path, explaining to your team why you believe in these values is important to obtain credibility. People are less likely to do something if they only know what to do, slightly better at doing the same thing if you explain how to do it, but they become real partners to achieve a common goal when they understand why they are asked to do something and how this can have a larger impact than themselves.

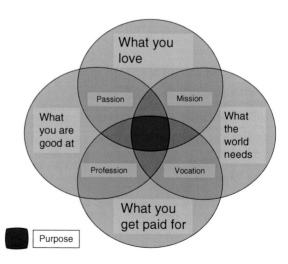

Fig. 55.1 Overlap of purpose

Reciprocity

Reciprocity is the capacity of being kind, even if this is not going to result on a direct outcome. In other words: paying it forward. When thinking about this principle, it is important that we keep in mind that giving is better than receiving when the gift is immaterial, for example, extending opportunities can be a form of giving. In some cases this can help increase your influence; however it has to be done ethically and it has to be genuine.

Authority

This principle refers not to have authority by speaking louder but of being an authority on a specific area. Being excellent clinically, since our training is to be surgeons, is of the highest importance on the path to leadership. Developing an area of expertise will give you authority and additionally the capacity to teach others.

Scarcity

This refers to knowing your value and making sure those around you understand it as well. The best example of this is in sales are the advertisements of "limited supply" or "limited time only." In surgical leadership this can be translated in time management. Understand you have control over your commitments and the value of your time. You need to balance the need to be available for your team, with the time that you invest in different projects.

Consensus

Uncertain people may look at the actions and decisions of others to determine their own. Before walking into a meeting, having the support of stakeholders or at least having them understand your point of view a priori can help with the amplification of your message and perhaps lead to better results.

Power Poses and Influence in Presence

Although confidence comes from within, there is some evidence that small interventions can affect how we feel about our capacity. In humans and other mammals, testosterone levels rise in individuals who hold situational power. Testosterone has

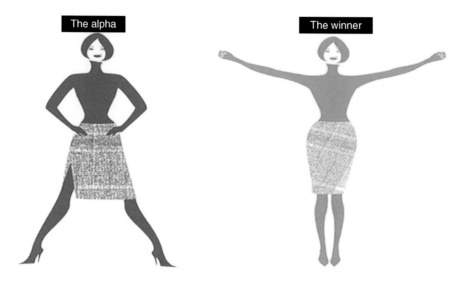

Fig. 55.2 Power poses: low power pose vs. high power pose

been shown to rise in anticipation of a competition and as a result of a winning and dropping following a defeat. Conversely cortisol has been associated with low power individual. Carney et al. [1] have shown decrease in cortisol level and increase in testosterone level in healthy volunteers that held power poses for 90 s or more. In the same study it was shown that cortisol level is higher in those individuals holding low power poses. Holding high power poses also has been associated with better performance in job interviews when performed prior to the challenge [2] (Fig. 55.2).

Power poses can be a quick fix to empower yourself and perform better under stress. However, building courage in difficult situations is a lifelong learning task. Being confident and seemingly confident might be connected, but they are not the same. Confident surgeons carry tools, not ordinances when it comes to human interactions. Being able to see the situations from a broad perspective without feeling defensive is part of having a growing mind-set.

References

1. Carney DR, Cuddy AJ, Yap AJ. Power posing: brief nonverbal displays affect neuroendocrine levels and risk tolerance. Psychol Sci. 2010;21(10):1363–8.
2. Cuddy AJ, Wilmuth CA, Yap AJ, Carney DR. Preparatory power posing affects nonverbal presence and job interview performance. J Appl Psychol. 2015;100(4):1286–95.

Suggested Reading

Archer J. Testosterone and human aggression: an evaluation of the challenge hypothesis. Neurosci Biobehav Rev. 2006;30(3):319–45.

Ayeleke RO, North N, Wallis KA, Liang Z, Dunham A. Outcomes and impact of training and development in health management and leadership in relation to competence in role: a mixed-methods systematic review protocol. Int J Health Policy Manag. 2016;5(12):715–20.

Moss SA, Wilson SG, Irons M, Naivalu C. The relationship between an orientation to the future and an orientation to the past: the role of future clarity. Stress Health. 2017;33(5):608–16.

Pillay R. The skills gap in hospital management: a comparative analysis of hospital managers in the public and private sectors in South Africa. Health Serv Manag Res. 2010;23(1):30–6.

Stavisky RC, Adams MR, Watson SL, Kaplan JR. Dominance, cortisol, and behavior in small groups of female cynomolgus monkeys (Macaca fascicularis). Horm Behav. 2001;39(3):232–8.

Yarbrough Landry A, Stowe M, Haefner J. Competency assessment and development among healthcare leaders: results of a cross-sectional survey. Health Serv Manag Res. 2012;25(2):78–86.

Part VI
Maintaining Your Health

Chapter 56
Work-Life Balance

Daniel Neff

Without a doubt, the first lecture I attended in medical school remains the most influential and important. During orientation week, we were visited by an alumnus who made our first lecture not about science or anatomy but about values. "You're entering onto a challenging and seductive path," he told us. He implored, "Don't be seduced."

Medicine is a field steeped in heroic myth and magic. Indeed, this was observed in the earliest societies in the powers bestowed upon the proverbial witch doctor or medicine man. Illness came as a supernatural villain visited upon its victims. At first, supernatural power was reflexively invoked to fight it. While Galen and others gifted us with the first scientific framework of medicine, our sociocultural role and own internal ethics have thankfully not yet fully relegated us to mere technicians.

We, and our patients, continue to labor under the presumption that what we do is particularly noble and meaningful. That was half the reason I found myself in medicine to begin with: to have the assurance I was making a meaningful contribution in this world, that I was working on something larger than myself. This belief that we cling to, that our work is meaningful and important, can be our salvation and our curse.

Putting aside the crude stereotypes of the detached physician "playing god" with power of life and death over others, there is a far more subtle and dangerous threat to those of us with good conscience. Self-sacrifice can become an unholy mortification when elevated above all else. We can in essence become possessed by our work. It is all too easy to be seduced by this "higher calling" and become neglectful of other areas of our lives. When we fall victim to this trap we risk destroying ourselves. I can do no better to elucidate the perils we face, and how real this threat is, than to recount my memory of what my lecturer told me.

D. Neff, MD
Department of Psychiatry and Human Behavior, Sidney Kimmel Medical College, Thomas Jefferson University, Philadelphia, PA, USA

© Springer International Publishing AG, part of Springer Nature 2018
K. Yoon-Flannery et al. (eds.), *A Surgeon's Path*,
https://doi.org/10.1007/978-3-319-78846-3_56

Imagine you've had a long day at work. You come home. The house is a mess, the yard work needs doing, the kids are clamoring for dinner, and you haven't even thought about your laundry. Your spouse has grown increasingly distant and unaffectionate. You'd like to share more with him or her, but let's face it, they just wouldn't understand. Besides, telling them how much you invest in work will only compound their frustration that you're short-changing your family. You've promised you were going to make time for visiting the in-laws but just can't seem to find it. Now, are you eager to rush home? Or, like many, wouldn't you prefer to stay at work that extra hour? After all, there are important things to be done. You work hard, all the nurses and patients think you're "just the best doctor, you really care," and most importantly they tell you this. Indeed, when working, you feel like that ancient witch doctor or priest, a figure revered and praised. Before long you're spending more and more time at work. You begin to resent your family for not appreciating you the way your staff and patients do. Can't they see how important you are? How can they think that their petty needs and problems compare to the awesome struggle with life and death you wage, and all too frequently win. So your anniversary rolls around, and you come up with the third lame dinner date in a row, resenting the responsibility all the while. And the in-laws? You take an extra shift at work when you could have relied on a colleague. After all, you know you'll do it better, and don't the patients deserve the quality of care that only you can provide. How can your family be so selfish and unappreciative?

A patient tells you you're her favorite doctor; you made that diagnosis everyone else missed. Young students revere you, and a hush comes over the OR as you step into the room. You've got the lowest complication rate in your practice, and you've published more articles than all the senior faculty in your department. Medical students backstab and sabotage each other for the opportunity to join one of your cases and retract for 15 h just in the hopes that you'll write them a letter. You are the captain of all you survey and a titan among your peers.

In as few words as possible: get over yourself. *This* is not who you wanted to be. I hope. You became a doctor not to become some monstrous demigod. Besides, etymologically a demigod is reciprocally a demi-man. The more godlike you find yourself becoming in your own mind, the more divine your work, the less human you necessarily become.

The crucial concern for all physicians in this matter is that the seductive power of positive regard and praise is easily underestimated. Over time it accumulates, and each concession in favor of work draws one further from life. At first blush, it may not seem obvious that work is antithetical to life. Nevertheless, philosophy, psychoanalysis, and even religion have all recognized the essential apposition of work and death against play and life. One needs to look no further for human awareness of this fact than the biblical creation myth of Adam that imagines a fall from endless play to a life of mortality and toil. When we consistently choose work, no matter how rewarding, over life, we mortgage parts of ourselves at decreasingly favorable interest rates.

What at first starts as invaluable praise for small self-sacrifice can lead to further self-compromise. As we have less and less to give outside of work to our families and ourselves, we are at risk of always chasing that next fix in the surest place we can get it. Alas, the law of diminishing returns rules over this process. At the end, we risk becoming that ghost of a doctor who prefers rounding at 4 AM with our residents to catching our kid's school play or recital. I ask again: "Is this who you wanted to become?"

As with stress management, prevention is the order of the day. To guard against this fate we must be aware of the dangers and alert for warning signs. When you notice yourself spending that extra hour at work, ask, "Is it *really* for the patients, or am I doing this to avoid something else?" When your relationship with your spouse becomes distant, do you retreat further into work or refocus on your marriage? When you haven't had a vacation in 2 years, is it because no one can really cover you or because you're afraid of being alone with your family? These are the questions we must be prepared to ask ourselves if we wish to remain healthy and spiritually alive. Whatever miracles we think we might be working for our patients, selling off our souls and destroying ourselves is not a compromise we have to make.

When we find ourselves giving way to the temptation to neglect ourselves and our larger lives outside of work, we will all be faced with a choice. Perhaps the greatest challenge will be recognizing that it is in fact a choice. You can choose to persistently and insistently choose your work over yourself and your family. In fact, you were likely trained to do so. This is not sustainable. The very phrase work-life balance is somewhat misleading. More accurate would be work-life exchange. One can either live to work or work to live. No matter how noble or meaningful the work, we must always endeavor to fulfill our first responsibility to ourselves and our families: to live.

Acknowledgment   Dedicated to Robert Brent, MD.

Chapter 57
Stress Management

Daniel Neff

Major transitions in the career path of rising physicians will bring increases in both privileges and responsibilities. In navigating these transitions through college, medical school, and residency training, most physicians will have become well acquainted with stress and coping strategies to manage. Unfortunately, many of the most readily adopted short-term coping strategies are prone to prove disastrous over the course of a physician's career. A mature and successful strategy to manage stress begins with proper evaluation of basic questions: What is stress? What does it mean? What causes it? What are good responses to it?

Stress, defined for our purposes, is the psychological appraisal of physiologic cues including increased heart rate, vasomotor tone, muscle tension, respiration, and other hallmarks of sympathetic activation. Such sympathetic activation marshals the body's resources to respond to challenges in the environment. The psychological appraisal of these cues serves functions beyond immediate response itself. When challenging situations arise, this appraisal system produces saliency that can be used for learning. An organism can learn both how to avoid stressful situations and how to respond when they occur.

Physicians, ego-strong masters of repression, often ignore these opportunities for learning in their commitment to career advancement and patient care. We can hardly be faulted for this state of affairs. The entire process of physician development is intrinsically challenging, sometimes maliciously so, and requires all who pursue it to deny, ignore, and negate their stress should they choose to continue. Only the most adept at this process progress through MCATs, shelf and USMLE exams, the match, and residency. Small wonder that we find a group that denies stress, persists in its presence, and perceives personal failure when their defenses against it fail.

D. Neff, MD
Department of Psychiatry and Human Behavior, Sidney Kimmel Medical College,
Thomas Jefferson University, Philadelphia, PA, USA

© Springer International Publishing AG, part of Springer Nature 2018   275
K. Yoon-Flannery et al. (eds.), *A Surgeon's Path*,
https://doi.org/10.1007/978-3-319-78846-3_57

Stress, properly understood, is a crucial informational tool not be ignored or taken lightly. As such, stress management for the physician often begins with stress recognition, acknowledgment, and acceptance. Having spent years being told, "Pain is weakness leaving the body," physicians have to unlearn shame at feeling stressed. Instead, when stress is acknowledged, it can provide the necessary signal for physicians to reevaluate their decisions, workload, and responsibilities and take alternative action. Those who ignore these cues are apt to find themselves ultimately overwhelmed and unhappy, hoist on their own petard. As we often tell our patients, "an ounce of prevention is worth a pound of cure." While not all stress needs to be fled, and indeed a minimal amount of stress can be healthy, it must be taken seriously and included in decision-making long before it has the opportunity to take root and fester.

Young physicians noticing stress might make a host of reasonable decisions. They might change course, picking that other specialty or rebalancing commitments and responsibilities. Should they opt to continue on the same path, they can adopt mitigation strategies and design safety valves to prevent a proverbial "boiling over." For those who struggle to even notice stress, multiple strategies can prove effective in restoring this skill. While outside the purview of this chapter, scheduled stress inventories and self-check-ins along with mindfulness can be indispensible tools. Stress and its more noxious cousin burnout are most damaging when they are left to continue ignored, denied, and uninterrupted.

What then does our intrepid young physician do when stress is noticed, acknowledged, and accepted? Rather than engage in the fantasy that stress can be entirely managed *away*, like a demon to be exorcised, physicians can endeavor to manage stress *in*. Responsible mitigation strategies begin with appreciating that stress is inevitable, acceptable, and appropriate. Like industrial pollution, planning for stress as a necessary by-product of productive activity allows us to regularly address and control it. Put simply, stress is best handled before a crisis occurs.

Successful stress mitigation strategies will vary from person to person. Regular and planned activities that restore our sense of efficacy and well-being are among the most helpful. These range from musical performance, exercise, yoga, meditation, and pleasure reading to time with family and friends. What these activities share in common is that they provide an opportunity for a change of mental state from persistent outward problem-solving to directed activity with inward focus. Without returning to this mental state, physicians are prone to lose their sense of self and efficacy, likely the very things that drew them to medicine in the first place.

One of the peculiar challenges facing physicians that produces a great deal of stress is one I first identified during my residency. The principal problem arises from a jarring transition in basic life currencies. Throughout medical education, which extends later in life compared to peers, our primary currency for barter and basic problem-solving is time. Indeed, much of the system of medical education is based on the assumption that medical student time is cheap and to be spent liberally. As such, when physicians arrive at challenges, their first impulse is to spend time to solve them. Indeed, up until this point, their time *is* cheap. However, as one transitions out of residency, time comes into an increasingly short supply. As time becomes scarcer, physicians who do not account for its transition from their primary resource will be at risk of spending it foolishly. Failure to adapt to a new time economy can result in tremendous stresses and produce great frustration. When we can no longer solve problems simply by allotting more time, we have to learn an entirely new problem-solving economy. Those who can adapt and begin to see time as a scarce asset with convertible monetary and other values are likely to better manage problems and mitigate stress.

In managing stress and time, young physicians face another somewhat unique challenge: learning to say "no." Medical education often extorts our propensity for repression and agreeableness. As a result, physicians first starting out have been trained to always say yes, submit to hierarchy, and "be a good team player." This self-sacrificial ethos can be toxic when taken to an extreme, and this is nowhere more common in medicine than the surgical fields. Physicians can hardly be good team players when they are overwhelmed, overworked, frustrated, and neglecting basic self-care. Remediation and practice in basic assertiveness skills are often essential to prevent and manage stress. An ability to "stand up for oneself" is not to be derided as selfishness but instead praised and reinforced. Indeed, if doctors cannot even effectively advocate for themselves, they will simultaneously fail to advocate for their patients.

In the final analysis, stress management might be quickly summarized as something "not worth getting stressed about." Instead, a mature approach to stress will focus on its inevitability and avoid viewing it as a matter of personal strength or weakness. Planning for stress and making its evaluation and management a routine component of preventative self-care presents the best mitigation strategy. Intentionally adopting healthy habits, including self-advocacy, should form the basis of this strategy for all physicians.

Chapter 58
Burnout

Marc Neff

This is a topic near and dear to my heart. Let me share with you some personal history. Over the past 3 years, my life has been a crucible. I have gone through death of my mother, separation and divorce, estrangement from my kids, change in living situation, change in employment, health issues including treatment for TB exposure with isoniazid, a recertification exam, multiple malpractice cases, and identity theft. Nonetheless was the constant pressure of work, patients, on-call responsibilities, new EHR computer system, training new staff, and teaching residents. Suffice it to say, I know a thing or two about burnout. I have read a gammit of books on grit, self-help, and positive psychology. The lessons I have learned would be a whole book by itself. In this chapter, I'm going to focus on an important underlying thread, burnout.

Physician burnout is only now starting to become a popular topic. It has long been looked upon as a sign of weakness to say you are tired, need a break, need a nap, or want to quit. Sadly, that culture is the breeding ground for mental, physical, emotional, and spiritual exhaustion that has real consequences in our lives as surgeons. Take a moment and do a quick google search, and you'll see that our career choice carries with it a higher addiction rate, suicide rate, and divorce rate, not something our faculty mentor told us back in medical school when we were choosing a career in surgery.

Let me start by asking some questions common to burnout.

Do you feel like you are tired? Wake up in the morning feeling like you got enough sleep? Feel like you have piles of mail you will never get to at home? In the office? Do you have any real hobbies? Any "me" time? Is your desk clean at the end of the day? Do you have a break for lunch? Do you spend any real time with your family? Do you find yourself snapping at people in office? In the OR? While driving

M. Neff, MD, FACS, FASMBS
Center for Surgical Weight Loss, Jefferson Health New Jersey, Cherry Hill, NJ, USA

to and from work? Do you need a drink to unwind? Do you find yourself feeling bitter? Unsympathetic? Unfocused? Do you schedule a conference just to get away? Do you ever get to exercise? What do you do to distress?

This list of questions seems silly, especially to the average resident, but they are real warning signs. Stress that is prolonged (work pressures, family pressures, relationship pressures) eventually gets to everyone. No one has infinite endurance. Eventually, you end up in a detached and empty state. That is burnout. It is when the stress of the daily grind continues so long, that you end up withdrawing from interpersonal interactions with family, colleagues, and friends. One of my favorite quotes that applies perfectly here is "You can't pour from an empty cup."

So why are surgeons so vulnerable? Because we are overachievers. We had to be to become surgeons. We had to work incredibly long hours, often sacrificing sleep, meals, friends, and family events. We have to take on incalculable workloads, do research, and take exams, and our goal is that we have to accomplish everything perfectly. And somehow, we know internally that we have to balance that with our life outside the hospital. It's a race. And the burned out surgeon feels like that are running on a treadmill and has no clue how to make it stop. If the race never ends, eventually every runner becomes tired. Chronic stress leads to exhaustion, cynicism, detachment, and true physical ailments.

Burnout is very real. It is like a chronic disease. The feelings of learned helplessness have been studied in dogs. The dog trapped in a cage given low-voltage electric shocks learns to ignore the shocks. Even when the cage door is opened, they don't rush to leave it because the shocks no longer register. The dogs become withdrawn, depressed, and physically sick. That is burnout. You or your colleague may be that very dog that has learned it can do nothing to avoid the shocks and has just become apathetic.

Our career as surgeons is full of challenges. Learning to recognize your own burnout (or your colleagues) and where to go to for help is just another. Sometimes, it is completely appropriate and infinitely valuable to check in with yourself, look yourself in a mirror, recognize your own needs, and then stop, rest, and fill your own gas tank before anyone else's and to put yourself first.

Suggested Reading

Phil Harley. Beating Burnout-Physician Heal Thyself. A guide for busy, tired, and stressed doctors. Brain Solutions. 2016.

Chapter 59
Diet and the Surgeon

Marc Neff

You've made it to completing a residency. You are the surgical attending. The embodiment of everything you ever wanted to be. You have the authority to take people to the operating room, put a knife to their body, and command a crew of six in a 15 × 15 foot room in their medical treatment. But I forgot to eat breakfast, the most important meal of the day.

Yes, we all forget it, because we weren't taught this in residency, the importance of eating right. Bad eating habits were everywhere in residency: snacks at the nursing station that are filled with chocolate and covered with powdered sugar; gifts from our patient that we feel we must eat because we earned it; greasy hours; old food we left in the call room before the case started; starving ourselves all day long because we don't need to take the time to eat (it's a sign that we are weak); and not eating because we have too much to do. The list goes on and on. But, the conclusion is we spend our residency focused on learning how to eat poorly. We don't learn to pack our lunches, how to meal prep, how to read labels, and how to plan out our upcoming busy office or OR day, and what happens is we make ourselves sick.

It happens slowly at first. A few pounds here and there. Less exercise because we have someplace to be. We can't be sweaty or out of breath for rounds or that important meeting. We can't be late to office hours. We can't take time out for ourselves. Then, if we are lucky, a fellow doctor makes a comment. We get some labs drawn after the prescription sitting in our pocket for months. We find that our cholesterol is elevated. Maybe it's our HgbA1c. We try to eat low fat for a few days. It's too hard to make our lunch. We miss dinner because of a late case. There are only a few minutes between cases so we grab a slice of pizza because a salad takes too long to make and too long to eat. And then, the sad truth is that we can't eat like we are in our 20s when we are in our 30s, 40s, and 50s.

M. Neff, MD, FACS, FASMBS
Center for Surgical Weight Loss, Jefferson Health New Jersey, Cherry Hill, NJ, USA

© Springer International Publishing AG, part of Springer Nature 2018
K. Yoon-Flannery et al. (eds.), *A Surgeon's Path*,
https://doi.org/10.1007/978-3-319-78846-3_59

I'm as guilty of it as the next person. Now, over 15 years since residency, I'm 60 pounds heavier, I prefer to take the elevator to the third floor than the stairs because I don't want to be out of breath when I get there, my back hurts after a long case, and my cholesterol is elevated. How can I expect to enjoy the 30-year surgical career I've always hoped for if I can't start taking care of the body I've been given like I encourage my patients to do?

So, here's the advice. Meal prep. Take a day. Sunday afternoon or evening. Wednesday evening. Take 2 h for yourself. Buy some protein. Chicken works fine. Get some vegetables. Buy some fruit and get some Tupperware. Meal prep some lunches for yourself. Make your own Bento box that will keep for 3 or 4 days. Do it twice a week if need be. Make different things each week. Variety is the spice of life. Go to the supermarket. Buy some healthy snacks. Take the time to read the label. Look at the calories, carbohydrates, fat, and salt intake. Plant some of these healthy snacks in your desk. In your OR locker. In your lab coat. Bring in fruit and/or vegetables with hummus to your long office hours. Put them in your kitchen. Snack on them first. Find a drink you like. Keep water with you as well as your coffee. Don't live your life dehydrated convincing yourself that you don't have the time to find a bathroom to urinate in.

Life as a surgical attending is overwhelming. It's the whole purpose of this book. But you can't expect to make it through the rest of your career if the fuel you put into your body is junk. Eventually, you'll end up as sick as your patients or even worse. If you eat better, you will feel better. You will be more productive. You will have more endurance. You will have the energy after the long day, to have some left to spend with your spouse, kids, partner, or family. We aren't taught so much to take care of ourselves in residency, but you need to as an attending. You aren't in your 20's anymore.

Chapter 60
When Is It a Good Time to Have a Baby?

Kahyun Yoon-Flannery

I remember the discussion I had with my mother-in-law at dinner when we were discussing my medical school admission news. My attorney husband and I had been married for almost 3 years already and were happily adjusted to our married life, managing it along with our professional lives, his as an attorney and mine as a researcher at a medical school. I had always vocalized my wish to become a physician, but my guess is that the news came as a surprise to some of our extended family members since we had seemed pretty stable. I told them that it would take 4 years to complete just the medical school part of it. Well, what about residency? What about internship? It wouldn't take more than 3–4 years, I assured them. And I remember my exact words to my mother-in-law: "Don't worry, mom, only surgery would take at least 5 years, and I'm definitely *not* doing surgery."

It took me less than 3 months of my first year of medical school to realize I wanted to be a surgeon. After classes and in between studying for many exams, I shadowed many physicians: pediatricians, emergency room physicians, family medicine doctors, and finally surgeons. After shadowing a surgeon and experiencing what it was like to be in the operating room, I had to swallow my words and tell everyone that I indeed wanted to be a surgeon, 5–7 long years, even after the 4 years of medical school. We knew we wanted to have a family, but it became unclear to me as to when would be the ideal time to attempt it. Looking around to the very few female physicians, let alone surgeons, it seemed that having a baby at all might not even be within our realm of possibilities as a family. I didn't really have a choice, and I moved forward with my career aspirations.

After two pre-clinical years and the first clinical year rotating through the "big four," surgery, internal medicine, OB/GYN, and pediatrics, my mind was solidified. I set my sub-internship rotations during my fourth year in medical school all for either general surgery or surgical subspecialty rotations. And I sat down with my

K. Yoon-Flannery, DO, MPH
Sidney Kimmel Cancer Center, Jefferson Health New Jersey, Sewell, NJ, USA
e-mail: kahyun.yoon-flannery@jefferson.edu

© Springer International Publishing AG, part of Springer Nature 2018
K. Yoon-Flannery et al. (eds.), *A Surgeon's Path*,
https://doi.org/10.1007/978-3-319-78846-3_60

283

husband finally to have "the discussion." Should we try to have this baby before I start my residency? It certainly wasn't easy, but I finally became pregnant after many visits to the OB/GYN and specialty offices. My daughter, first of four, came in November of my fourth year as a medical student. It was quite the attraction for me to show up to all my general surgery interviews, visibly and fully pregnant. My match day came a few months after that, thankfully with good news, and I was able to finish out my last year as a medical student graduating on time with my classmates.

As a female surgeon, especially after having three kids and with one currently on the way, I often get asked questions about motherhood from residents, interns, and medical students. Is it possible to have a family if I want to be a surgeon? I find it very discouraging to hear from some of my medical students that they had been given the usual talk "If you want any kind of a life that involves having a decent family, surgery is *not* a good option for you." Yes, there is no doubt that my years of training as a general surgeon, then moving forward with a surgical subspecialty with fellowship training, were difficult and long. I missed many special days for my family, including my children's first days of school and their birthdays, due to work obligations. My husband who also has a demanding career as an attorney, and now as a partner at a firm, is and has always been the backup person for every emergency despite his own difficult hours.

So you may be wondering, it doesn't seem really possible to maintain a good career as a surgeon and maintain a family. No, but it is possible. I had my first child, my daughter, as a fourth year medical student. Despite going on my interviews pregnant, the fourth year was the easiest year to be pregnant, especially towards the end, after the match. I had my second, Leo, as a second year general surgery resident. That was certainly much more difficult, with demanding call schedules, and trying to navigate through my own deficiencies and uncertainties as a junior resident, while trying to fight the others' perception of a *pregnant* surgical resident. I would probably not recommend being pregnant as a second year! My third, Max, was born in the month between my general surgery graduation and the start date of my fellowship training. I was pregnant again as a chief resident, where although the cases could be long and more technically challenging, I had more flexibilities (as flexible as an inflexible surgical resident schedule can be) arranging my cases. I am currently pregnant in my first year out as an attending, and that certainly has had its own issues. No more post call days to schedule your obstetrics visits and having a discussion with a patient to schedule a surgery around your due date has certainly brought on its own challenges.

I have also witnessed a lot of my colleagues and mentors who decide to put off their family plans until they complete their formal training. If we say that the average person goes to medical school immediately after college and spends 4 years as a medical student, by the time they start residency training, they are looking at 26–27 years of age. Add 5–6 years of general surgery training alone, you are looking at mid-30s. And if you have fellowship training, you add a few years on top of that. I had someone tell me, well you don't want to have a baby during your first year out as an attending when you're setting up your practice! Ok fine, so you wait another 2–3 years. You are well into your 40s before you may realize the clock had been ticking all along and now you are requiring fertility assistance. And even if you are successful with your first pregnancy and delivery, most people would want at least a sibling for their first child. And the same road lies ahead, probably a little bit more challenging, because of course you are becoming older.

I did not write the previous paragraph to highlight the difficult challenges in becoming a parent as a surgeon. I wrote it to highlight the fact that there is never a *perfect* time to have a baby. Surgical training is very difficult, with many road blocks in the way, but if family life is truly what you desire, it can certainly co-exist. You can have a baby during your training, and you will still manage to become a wonderful surgeon. What you have to remember is that no matter when you do it, you have to realize you may not be present for every single important milestone. I was on call the day of my daughter's second birthday. Twenty-four hours of call. I left the house at 5 am as I always did, and as I did not want to wake her up, I did not get to hug or kiss my daughter on the day of her birthday. It broke my heart. As I was making rounds in the middle of the night for the umpteenth time, looking at my list of patients, I burst into tears in the hall. Not one of those moments where there are some tears welling up in your eyes and you scare them away, but one of those ugly sobbing moments. But I picked myself up. I finished my rounds, and my call, and took care of all my patients. And I went home the next day, and we pretended the next day was her birthday. We blew out the candles on her Bubble Guppies cake, just as she wanted. She never remembered I missed her birthday. I still remember that I did miss it, but my daughter would never know it.

Having a surgical career certainly presents a challenging road ahead, but if having a family is an aspiration, you should not compromise your career or your family plans. There will never be a perfect time to plan everything as a surgeon, but if you are lucky enough to have support alongside the career you always wanted, you will figure out how to navigate through the challenges life throws at you. We are born problem solvers. We can do anything.

Chapter 61
Social Media and Your Professional Presence Online

Christian Jones and Elliott R. Haut

Introduction

Surgery is a team sport. Surgeons can and must rely on outstanding nurses, technicians, administrators, colleagues, and other specialists to deliver the best possible patient care. This community of professionals allows each individual to confront the challenges and tasks for which they are best equipped. While self-reliance and individual autonomy are stereotypical hallmarks of surgeons, a network of healthcare providers encourages ongoing education and personal and interpersonal growth.

Additionally, patient and community outreach, once the domain of primary care providers, is now the standard of care in numerous surgical specialties—oncology, bariatrics, trauma, and vascular. Many surgeons find satisfaction and meaning in engaging current and potential patients in medical conversations. Similarly, patients and patient advocates discover outstanding practitioners through public or semipublic engagement and further their own understanding of illnesses and treatments.

Long ago, these engagement efforts were limited to individual surgeons, institutions, and local medical societies. The rapid adoption of online communities, both general and specialized, led to the widespread adoption of Internet physician profiles and social media interactions. These tools are invaluable to the young surgeon's professional and personal development, and though appropriate caution is warranted, investing the time to manage an online presence can be worthwhile.

C. Jones, MD, MS, FACS (✉) · E. R. Haut, MD, PhD, FACS
Division of Acute Care Surgery, Department of Surgery, Johns Hopkins University School of Medicine, Baltimore, MD, USA
e-mail: on-call@christianjones.md; ehaut1@jhmi.edu

The Internet Is Forever

The recurring theme of this chapter, and the major warning regarding use of the Internet for professional activity (or any activity), is *the Internet is forever*.

Forever.

No, really. FOREVER.

The picture of you during medical school with a red Solo cup in your hand, your eyes slightly out of focus, and your attire "not quite appropriate" was deleted within 30 min of your friend's post, but it's still out there. In fact, it may have been accessed and used as an example of "unprofessional behavior" in a scholarly work suggesting physicians should avoid the Internet altogether. It could be available for download as an online supplement to the paper.

It doesn't matter that the cup was filled with orange juice, your eyes were bleary due to being open all night preparing for your neurosciences final, and you dressed like that because it was *ridiculously* hot. The post is still there, even though you hoped deleting it would solve the problem. *The Internet is Forever* and appearances matter.

This is not to discourage posting and participation, quite the opposite. Avoiding the appearance of impropriety is important, but open and honest discussion of the personal and professional lives of physicians delivers public engagement and identification of the surgeon as a "real person." Unfortunately, even "real people" can make mistakes. We suggest a momentary pause accompanied by a bit of thought may prevent needless suffering.

Online Ratings

Search for your name, maybe with "surgeon," your degree, or your city. Use the generic Internet search engine of your choice. Don't try to get more specific—this will be one way patients and other members of the public will try to find out information about you. You'll likely find the first several results include physician profile and rating web sites like Vitals, Healthgrades, and WebMD, physician communities like Doximity, and perhaps institutional or professional association profile pages. You may identify a few problems; for instance, (CJ) still gets several hits referring to providers with the same name in other cities and practicing different specialties (and not all of their ratings are positive). You could, on the other hand, have a relatively unique name (ERH) and not have this problem at all.

Public ratings of physicians are in high demand, and those that exist are subjective, suffer from recall biases and other sampling problems, and are quickly identified by potential patients who understand quite well the implications of a one-star rating for their future surgeon. Most allow you to "claim" your profile, add information to it, and even respond to or request the removal of poor reviews. However, there are not definitive leaders in this field; even review sites not specific to doctors (like Yelp and Angie's List) have developed the ability to "rate your surgeon," and keeping up to date with all the profiles available is likely not the best use of your time.

Instead, cultivation of a "professional profile" via your institution or a surgical association like the American College of Surgeons (ACS) or the Association for Academic Surgeons (AAS) will appear reliable and useful to the public. An added benefit is that these official profiles are often given preference as results in search engines, appearing before less reputable sites. Similarly, U.S. News & World Report partners with Doximity to provide accurate physician profiles, ones that tend to be among the most reputable and most easily found with a simple search. "Claiming" and completing these profiles provides the opportunity not only to make undesirable (or unaffiliated) results end up further down a search result page and thus less likely to be accessed but will also help provide the public with accurate objective information about you and your practice.

Physician Communities

Physician-specific web sites provide some level of apparent "professional privacy." Doximity and Sermo confirm physician identities prior to approval of accounts and claim to function as "digital physician lounges" for medical and social discussions in an era in which physical physician lounges are becoming more rare. Surgical associations have similar offerings, such as the ACS Communities, that are accessible only to members. Each of these sites includes comments about the latest literature, practice patterns, and nonmedical topics such as politics. Expected etiquette in such communities, like the rest of the Internet, varies widely, and new members are strongly advised to "lurk" or listen into conversations to establish the norms in any given corner of the network before actively posting your own content or opinions.

Furthermore, despite the purportedly closed nature of these communities and others like "private" groups on Facebook, users are once again reminded that *the Internet is Forever*. Professional conduct is encouraged, despite its occasional absence depending on the community. Moreover, patient privacy must be strictly maintained, a delicate balance when attempting to discuss a specific case, whether teaching or requesting advice. Since *the Internet is Forever*, even comments that do not directly include protected health information can be combined with timestamps, public records, and media coverage to violate patient confidentiality. The safest approach is to never post patient-specific information, radiology images, or photographs.

Blogs and Microblogs

The ease of publishing educational material to the Internet rapidly led to the rise of Free Open Access Medical education, commonly referred to as "FOAM" or "#FOAMed". This includes personal and corporate blogs like Medscape and KevinMD but also short-form items posted to Twitter, Facebook, Instagram, and other social media sites. These "microblogs" encourage community sharing and feedback and may be intentionally geared toward engaging the public, patients, or other physicians. In addition to the posts about medical topics including clinical patient care and research, the communities limiting the traditional hierarchy allow open discussion of social issues in medicine, like diversity, burnout, work-life balance, and building families. They also encourage multidisciplinary discussion; we routinely benefit from conversations with specialists in all areas of surgery, as well as internists, palliative care physicians, public health experts, nurses, pharmacists, patient organizations, and emergency medical services (EMS) providers from around the world.

Like physician-only communities, social media sites require adaptation to normal expectations. Get to know the sites and their content before actively posting. Professionalism is important, even when having a public discussion with friends and partners; what you may have meant in a joking manner may not be received in the same way. A plethora of guides for physicians and surgeons about "Getting Started with Twitter" is easily found with a simple Internet search.

The Internet Is (Still) Forever (We Told You It Was Recurring.)

Patient privacy protection is the obvious corollary to the aforementioned concerns about physician "professionalism." As noted above, even otherwise innocuous information can be combined with other data to determine specifics about a particular patient or operative case. A post about "massive blood loss" or "just finishing a huge, tough case with Dr. XXXXX" may be seen by the patient's family, leading to unnecessary anguish. In a famous example of public sharing of "nonidentifiable" patient information, an emergency department patient died on a "reality" television show. Despite care to blur his features, the patient's family easily identified him based on the location and circumstances and was understandably distraught. Regardless of intention or legal ramifications, harm is apparent. Don't post about patients—*the Internet is Forever.*

Takeaways

- *The Internet is Forever.*
- Patients gather information about physicians—cultivate your online profile.
- Social media is a powerful tool for professional education and support.
- *The Internet is Forever.*

Chapter 62
Mindfulness

William D. Stembridge

I am convinced that I was asked to write this chapter based solely on the qualification of being the "least irate resident" in my program. While flattering, the observation is based mostly on a generally flat affect and quiet demeanor. Nevertheless, I gladly accepted the task based upon the following conditions:

- My thoughts may stand a remote chance of reducing the daily stress of even one surgery resident or staff member (even for one moment).
- I have learned a lot about myself from thinking through this topic and expounding.
- Any book my mentor Dr. Marc Neff touches is gold.
- I will distinctly enjoy looking back at this in 20 years for a good laugh.

With that stated, I will share a fact that will come as a surprise to those who know me from residency: that in my formative years I was quite a worrier. I abhorred failure and disappointment. I literally cried if I struck out in a little league baseball game. I had nightmares of getting in trouble at school in front of my friends. Getting a grade of less than an A was out of the question. My parents were not overbearing. They are quite the opposite, in fact, as they are very supportive to this day and were in no way to blame for my rather neurotic behavior at the time (although I know it must have worried them). I even received my first self-help book from my dad when I was about 12. It was titled *Don't Sweat the Small Stuff* by Richard Carlson. Even before I cracked the book open, I realized I needed to take it down a notch.

Since that time, I have slowly taught myself to go with the flow a little more, both outwardly and inwardly. I trust in the fact that almost all people battle some degree of similar conflict. With that in mind, the impressions expressed here are solely my own, formed over the course of 30-something years growing up and culminating in 5 years of general surgery residency, under the tutelage of some excellent surgeons

W. D. Stembridge, DO
Advanced GI Minimally Invasive and Bariatric Surgery, Anne Arundel Medical Center,
Annapolis, MD, USA

© Springer International Publishing AG, part of Springer Nature 2018
K. Yoon-Flannery et al. (eds.), *A Surgeon's Path*,
https://doi.org/10.1007/978-3-319-78846-3_62

with a wide breadth of attitudes and emotions. Anyone reading this knows that the situations encountered in the daily comings and goings of a general surgeon range from boring to utterly insane, with the two extremes typically separated by mere moments. As such, this chapter is written in a colloquial rather than a scientific light. Any humor is intended in a lighthearted manner but not to diminish the importance of remaining mindful, even when the going gets tough.

The Merriam-Webster Dictionary helped to eloquently condense the title of a chapter originally referred to as "How to avoid being the obnoxious surgeon who loses his mind and acts like an addled child every time something doesn't go his way" into a single word:

Mindfulness.

noun mind·ful·ness \ 'mīn(d)-fəl-nəs \
The practice of maintaining a nonjudgmental state of heightened or complete awareness of one's thoughts, emotions, or experiences on a moment-to-moment basis.

In keeping with the title of this book, there is no chapter in any surgery textbook that describes an objective technique for maintaining this simple but fleeting state (there is probably a good reason no such chapter exists, but we will give it a shot anyways). Yet surgeons, much to the despair of their fellow OR staff, floor nurses, administrators, residents, medical students, families, and, on unlucky days, pets, often battle with an absence of mindfulness on a nearly daily basis. Lapses in temper, judgment, and control not only offend those on the receiving end of the discussion but also waste time and resources, decrease staff and patient confidence, and generally give surgeons a bad name. We all trust that stories of surgeons flipping over Mayo stands, throwing instruments, or hurling obscenities in a completely unfettered way are a relic of the past. But even the smallest amount of passive-aggressive pushback from a single member of the surgical team can cause disruption.

I can firmly say that of all the surgeons I now know and have worked closely with, none are in fact bad people. None gains any satisfaction or enjoyment from being frustrated beyond the point of control in front of other professionals. None considers it macho or typical to become unwound during work. And this speaks loudly to the crux of the matter: being a general surgeon is an exceedingly stressful, high-stakes, low margin-for-error profession. Don't push the knot down tying that middle thyroid vein in a thyroidectomy? A patient develops a hematoma at home and loses the airway. The stapler misfires as you cross the splenic vessels? You've got a blood bath on your hands. Wait 12 hours too long to take that *Clostridium difficile* colitis patient to the OR? Sepsis too overwhelming to overcome. All are literal life-threatening/ending situations that happen not uncommonly in hospitals across the country and involve general surgeons. Your first case of the day doesn't go well; you don't like how that anastomosis turned out and the case took twice as long as expected. Better reboot because you've got four more to go! Only now the remaining patients will be upset they had to wait, the OR staff will have to undergo a full-shift change halfway through a case, and the anesthesiologist is griping about being out of crossword puzzles to do. Never mind the dozen patients on the floors, some awaiting test results or exam findings that necessitate an add-on operation, others waiting to be discharged once they tolerate lunch, and the rest languishing in hospital limbo. Oh, and the ED just called about a patient in bed 2 with severe abdominal pain and no work-up. You get the point, and if reading this makes you nervous and angry or does anything other than put a smile on your face, then you're probably at risk for a lapse in mindfulness.

So what can be done when these inevitable situations arise? Having brought much success in my adolescent years, I harkened back to Dr. Carlson's eloquent words in his aptly titled book *Don't Sweat the Small Stuff, and It's All Small Stuff.*

Well, a multiple patient triage event on trauma night call isn't small stuff, nor can I take a walk instead of addressing the mangled bodies dropped off by EMS! But alas, the saying isn't obsolete for surgeons, it's about sorting out what is deserving of sweat. Treating the unrestrained child who is short of breath: not small stuff; give it hell. A TICU nurse inadvertently calls during the work-up: small stuff and probably not deserving of a berating. Miss the late-night cafeteria opening: questionably not small stuff, especially if you've been on for 24 hours and missed two other meals under similar circumstances (pro tip: Trauma attendings love any excuse to order out food). Without plagiarizing Dr. Carlson's entire book, it's definitely worth reading for anyone who wants a proper and professional undertaking of the concept of mindfulness and stress management. There is much to learn about the ways surgeons, as ambitious and overachieving individuals, stand in their own paths. By taking a step back, it's possible not only to achieve more but to also enjoy the process.

So first, foremost, and most importantly, identify times when you are at risk of a lapse in mindfulness. Obviously this is quite hard; if you always did it you would already be mindful. Once you are in the mindful spirit, you will notice many triggers for becoming frustrated, mad, or ornery that would have otherwise been swept under the rug. Next, bite your tongue. I unanimously regret everything I've ever said in moments of negative emotion and duress. Or at least wished I could go back and reword them. Personally, I can't do much better than a short iteration of a prayer commonly referred to as the Serenity Prayer. Originally attributed to an evangelical preacher in Massachusetts named Reinhold Niebuhr in the 1930s and used tirelessly since, think:

Change the things that can be changed,
Accept those that cannot,
And have the wisdom to know the difference.

Finally, practice. Just like tying better knots or spending hours on the laparoscopy trainer, you can practice mindfulness. Identify each situation through the day and how you would have reacted had you not caught yourself. As you get better, you will probably start to notice more and more occurrences throughout the day.

Physicians are very well trained in making diagnoses. Unfortunately, knowing what personal battles should be fought is rarely understood in a 5–7-year residency to the degree that multiple endocrine neoplasms are. The following are some thoughts that I have jotted down in past weeks while further exploring this topic:

Around the Hospital

– Bad situations are going to happen to you, often. You're a general surgeon after all. Own that. You're the guy or gal everyone else wants to have around when things get gritty, because you deal with gritty situations day in and day out.
– Stress and loss of mindfulness don't always stem from high intensity or frantic times. Some of my most angry days of residency were spent in a quiet call room with nothing going on, brooding about how all my friends and families were enjoying their normal lives. This brooding mentality would often rear itself as discontentment and resent toward other people I interacted with that day, from the friends I was jealous of to the nurse who needed a Tylenol order.
– You'll get a consult so bizarre, so scary, that you don't even want to see the patient. Don't avoid the situation; lean into it. There is no use in distracting yourself from the inevitable and unknown. Granting yourself the authority and will to tackle any consult, problem, or operation is far more empowering than shying away from it. The most grizzled, salty, hardened surgeons I have ever operated with and would follow into the gates of hell still see cases that defy imagination. But they get through it.
– Ask for help. While we would like to do everything ourselves, other services exist for a reason. And they must learn a few tricks in those long medicine fellowships.
– We all know there are situations that truly do need to be addressed, sometimes even in a more aggressive way. Prepare yourself for these times and do so in a controlled and professional manner.

Among the Residents

– Residents are a team. Whether you love every other resident, would spend time out of the hospital with some, or hate all their guts, there is a special bond in residency. For 3–7 years, you act as the overworked, underpaid, rarely appreciated workhorses of the hospital. Nonphysician staff don't get it. Patients don't get it. Some attendings have even forgotten what it was like.
– Police your own residency. No matter what postgrad year, you should all be proud of each other and how your program is seen by the hospital. This doesn't mean best hair and makeup, most likely to make the hospital softball team, or most Tinder matches. It means most likely to be ready, knowledgeable, competent, and take the best care of the patients. This may mean tough love. The definition of tough love can be left to the discretion of individual programs, but most where I come from agree that you don't want to be on the receiving end of it.
– Hold each other accountable from within.

– When an outsider challenges your group, be prepared to politely stick up for one another. If an administrator, ancillary staff, or random person has a lapse in mindfulness and acts inappropriately toward your fellow resident, step in, calm the situation, and state that it will be taken care of by the residency program director. No one else gets to yell at you as a resident besides your seniors and attendings.
– As a resident, no patient will ever officially be yours, but treat every patient as if he or she is your only patient.
– When it comes to attendings, there is a difference between being right and being happy. You may do a laparoscopic cholecystectomy the way William Halsted himself would be proud of, but you'd also better be able to do it that way the attending you're scrubbed with wants it done.
– Prop each other up. Tell the ICU nurses how well the PGY-4 did sewing the anastomosis in the long case. Invite the intern into the OR for a few extra cases after she has been busting her tail on the floor all week.
– Don't be afraid to ask for help. Ask your buddy. Ask a senior. If you're really stuck, ask the chief. If hell is freezing over and zombies are invading the hospital, ask the program director. Don't make the wrong decision or miss an opportunity because you were too stubborn to ask for help.

Patient Care

– You don't *have to* make hard decisions every day. You *get to* make hard decisions every day and perform hard procedures. And present hard information, hard facts, and seasoned judgment to patients and families. Nearly every single decision to operate or not operate, stay laparoscopic, or open the abdomen, opt for palliative care or go for the cure, keep NPO or start a diet is one of *the* biggest decisions in that patient's day, week, year, and even life. You have earned the privilege to make these decisions many times over in a day.
– Since finishing residency, I've come to know the joys of patient calls from the answering service. There is no end to the breadth of thinking, wondering, absurdity, and sometimes utter disregard for time and sleep that come via the answering service. Rest assured, the patients aren't calling to be pests, and what may seem asinine is in fact a pressing, even stressful issue in his or her mind. I'm sure I sound the same way when I call AppleCare about my iPhone acting up.
– You'll make the wrong decision sometimes. There will be bad outcomes based on your actions. Patients may die. Your anastomoses will break down. You will feel bad. The patient, family, and staff will feel terrible. But the show must go on. There are other decisions to make and lives to affect.
– Don't be afraid to ask for help. Sometimes we get tunnel vision, especially on the most complicated cases. Ask someone else to take a look with you, help you out, and have a feel for the case.

At Home

- Try not to bring your work home with you. While tales of heroic ED thoracoto-mies or photos of foreign bodies removed precariously (HIPAA violations are also generally frowned upon) may make for top entertainment over a drink, your husband or wife and kids probably would rather talk about normal family topics.
- Be patient. Their day may not have been as high strung as yours. It may have been more high strung.
- When you're home, be a husband/wife, father/mother, and son/daughter above all else. Leave the surgeon stuff at work.
- Enjoy the happy and peaceful times with your family and friends, even if they are boring times. These are the times you'll remember when you're old, not your interesting case you presented for grand rounds.
- We are forced to raise our tolerances to stress to very high levels as a necessary aspect of the profession. As a result, we must be more cognizant of our stress levels creeping up, even if they aren't high enough to break. This will help you to balance the stress and cope with it when time permits.
- Ask for help. (Hint: This has been in every section, star it for the test.) If there is a topic at work that you aren't able to cope with on a personal level, talk to some-one about it. I don't mean hashing out why Mr. Jones is persistently hypona-tremic despite your interventions, but rather what to do when you get your first bad evaluation, you find out the scrub tech at work passed away, or your emo-tions are just too much.

Conclusion

In summary, be humble and be patient. The wisdom part will come. While being a surgery resident or attending may garner you the trust of your patients, the admira-tion of your friends, a well-deserved salary, or maybe just a lot of hours spent in the hospital, you're part of a *team* of *people* who take care of *people*. Our ER colleagues never invite us to their wilderness medicine conferences because we are pretty use-less without our teams (an OR, modern instruments, medications, endoscopic linear stapling devices, etc.). Your success as a physician, surgeon, family member, income earner, employee, or business owner and even as a patient one day depends on your interactions with these people. Being a surgeon isn't easy, and there are many things they don't teach you in residency, but a little mindfulness can go a long way.

Chapter 63
Divorce

Marc Neff

You spend your days running from office to hospital to operating room. You come home to hostility, disrespect, and dishonesty. You've tried the marriage counseling. You've tried reading helpful posts on Facebook and on other websites. You've spoken to your friends, family, and colleagues. You find yourself spending more time at the hospital to avoid conflict with your partner. Sounds familiar? The scope of this chapter will focus not on how you got to the point of considering a divorce but what you can expect over the next 2 years.

First, be prepared to spend a lot of money, *a lot of money*! As much as you might be thinking that this will be an amicable process, it won't be when complicated with lawyers. It won't become a battle, you might think. You are so wrong. Remember, you are getting divorced because you and/or your partner has emotionally withdrawn from the marriage. You have lost the connection, the trust, and the respect. Don't imagine for a second that it will all of a sudden return when the lawyers get involved. My divorce took over 2 years, and well over $150,000, and that's pretty good from what I hear of what it can turn into. Custody evaluators cost money. Every phone call/email to your lawyer and accountant costs money. And that doesn't include the money you will spend on alimony and child support. And it doesn't include the money spent on rebuilding your life with a new apartment or house, food, furnishings, clothes, and all the while you might be starting to spend money dating again.

Second, be prepared to spend (waste) a lot of time, *a lot of time*! It takes time to visit the lawyer; time to review documents from the lawyer; time to go to court; time to go to the bank and open new accounts; time to make phone calls to mortgage companies and life insurance companies and change addresses on all your important documents; time to get copies of everything; time to go to the counselor and work on yourself; time to spend with your kids; time to rebuild your life and self-respect; and time to start dating again. Also, you will spend a lot of time not utilizing

M. Neff, MD, FACS, FASMBS
Center for Surgical Weight Loss, Jefferson Health New Jersey, Cherry Hill, NJ, USA

© Springer International Publishing AG, part of Springer Nature 2018
K. Yoon-Flannery et al. (eds.), *A Surgeon's Path*,
https://doi.org/10.1007/978-3-319-78846-3_63

your time wisely, time that will be wasted thinking of why this happened and what you could have done or be doing differently, and time spent just staring at the bottom of your glass of scotch and/or at the four walls of your new living space.

Third, be prepared to go through one of the most stressful times in your life. If you have been through a malpractice case, then you know stress. With lawyers, depositions, and experts, the process is never ending and like a noose that slowly tightens. The divorce process is much the same. Almost daily there will be some aggravation, maybe an email from your soon-to-be ex, some family interaction or holiday or school event that you have to face, a document from your lawyer to review, and upcoming evaluation by some expert. Maybe it's a counseling session. It will consume your focus and challenge your balance and inner peace. You will have trouble sleeping and trouble eating healthy. You will have less patience for nonsense and start developing a short temper. And, if you are so unfortunate as to have to deal with a malpractice case at the same time, just schedule the appointment with the psychologist now. We are taught to be resilient and show grit when it comes to being a surgeon in the trauma bay or keeping focus during a lengthy operation, but this is unlike anything you can possible imagine. It won't be easy. It won't be a sprint. You have a "life sentence" with the person you married, and that doesn't end when you decide the marriage is over; the "fun" is just beginning.

Lastly, slow down. Take the time to look yourself in the mirror, what you could be doing differently. To be healthy, you need to focus on your physical, emotional, intellectual, and spiritual health. Most of us have maxed out on the intellectual. We often let the physical go by the way side during residency and attending hood. Few of us focus on the spiritual and next to none of us on the emotional. That is the one that is the most critical.

Last points of advice:

1. Be sure you really want this. It's going to be incredibly costly, distracting, time-consuming, and going to impact on your relationship with your kids.
2. Be sure you've tried everything else—read the books, done the counseling together and separately, tried reconnecting, tried date night, and tried to rekindle the love you once had for each other.
3. Have copies of every document and picture and possession, because anything you don't have in your office will likely not be returned to you if/when you leave the house.

Lastly, once the process is done, you will be happier than you have been in years and stronger than you can possibly imagine, with a mental toughness that enables you to face and conquer the next life challenge with relative ease. You will be a source of courage and compassion to your family and friends. Residents, nurses, and friends will come to you for advice. You will have a newfound sense of emotional maturity and mindfulness. You will learn what mistakes to avoid the second time around. You will be scarred, but stronger.

Chapter 64
Life as a Surgeon from a Spouse's Perspective

James J. Cavello, Peter M. Flannery, and Melissa Cartolano

This chapter is meant to provide some insight on what your partner may be feeling with regard to your profession and also provide some tips on how you can better manage your relationship with your significant other to keep your partnership strong. In this chapter, we will start with developing an understanding of the additional personal burdens your partner will take on given the demands of your profession and then go into some techniques that can be utilized to help the two of you stay on the same page and continue to help each other achieve your mutual professional/personal goals.

There is no way around it; you have a very demanding job from a time and effort perspective. Given the amount of energy that is expended working at this profession on a day-to-day basis, it can be very easy to lose sight of the additional burdens that your significant other bears given the demands of your job. To do this, however, could breed contention in your relationship. Because your profession will demand more of your time than the typical person, your personal life (and relationships) will be the place where that time is most likely made up. There will be holidays and parties that your partner will have to plan and execute alone because you may be on call; and, there will be many errands and chores that most couples tackle together that will disproportionately fall on your partner because you don't work "normal" business hours. One of the most important things you can do to keep your relationship strong is to not lose sight of these additional pressures that your significant other will take on. Simple acknowledgment of what your partner takes on for the

J. J. Cavello, MBA (✉)
Johnson & Johnson, Horsham, PA, USA

P. M. Flannery, Esq
Bisgaier Hoff, Haddonfield, NJ, USA
e-mail: pflannery@bisgaierhoff.com

M. Cartolano, MSN
Frankfurt, IL, USA

© Springer International Publishing AG, part of Springer Nature 2018   299
K. Yoon-Flannery et al. (eds.), *A Surgeon's Path*,
https://doi.org/10.1007/978-3-319-78846-3_64

both of you will go a very long way. Thank you's are a very easy (and yet remarkably underutilized) way to show your partner that you are cognizant of the additional tasks they have shouldered. Even if it is for something as simple as picking up the dry cleaning, the thank you will go a long way with your partner because they will know that you know and appreciate all they do for you.

When it is feasible for you to pick up the slack and help out with some of the more mundane tasks humans have to deal with, do it! You will have a partner that appreciates that you are taking what little free time you have pitching in to ensure your lives are running smoothly. Also, performing these sorts of gestures when they are possible will not be forgotten by your partner. In fact, it will help them continue to shoulder these burdens even when they are having a tough day because they will know that their partner cares about them, and if they could take on some of these demands, they would.

At the end of the day, if you want a solid foundation to build off of for your relationship, it starts with understanding and acknowledging the unique dynamic that surgeons rely on their partners for an awful lot outside of hospital. With this empathetic mindset informing your overall approach to your relationship, here are some tips you can utilize to help keep that relationship strong.

Before your fellowship begins, you should ascertain your typical hours, call schedule, required conferences, and other obligations for the fellowship and share this information with your significant other. Because a surgical fellowship is often an intense training program with few (if any) co-fellows to share the workload, your fellowship may be more demanding than your chief year in general surgery residency with respect to hours, call schedule, conferences, and other obligations. It is important that your significant other is aware of your obligations during fellowship, especially if your significant other had become accustomed to a less demanding schedule during your chief year of residency or is otherwise expecting a less demanding schedule because you are now nearing the end of your surgical training. In addition, because some rotations may require longer hours than others, you should provide your significant other with information regarding the typical hours for each rotation taking place during your fellowship so that he/she can plan accordingly. When ascertaining these typical hours, you should also take into account the location of each rotation because commuting times to and from these locations will affect your time away from home. To the extent you are able to do so in advance, you should also ascertain what out-of-town conferences you will be required to (or are recommended to) attend during your fellowship. This will not only allow you to make advanced arrangements for yourself to attend the conferences, but it will also allow your significant other to make arrangements to attend with you or to arrange for assistance with childcare and/or other household matters while you are away.

For those with families, it is also important to balance the needs of your family against the demands of your fellowship or your position overall. Although it may be difficult, if not impossible, to change your work hours, call schedule, or conference commitments, you should try to limit your participation in voluntary events such as "rep" dinners or networking events (especially if they are not relevant to your practice area) so that you can spend that time with your family. It's better to have a simple meal with your kids than to have steak with a stranger trying to sell you something. In addition, although your significant other will likely take on the primary parenting role, it is important for you to communicate/coordinate with your significant other regarding the scheduling of practices, games, recitals, school open houses/conferences, etc., so that you can participate in your children's lives outside the home whenever possible. Oftentimes, due to the substantial amount of time that a surgeon spends outside the home, a significant other takes on a "single parent" or "military spouse" mentality and schedules events without you, assuming that you are not available. By becoming actively involved in the scheduling of these events, you will be able to participate when you can and not "miss out" on important milestones. Furthermore, even though your significant other will likely be responsible for most household tasks, you should take responsibility for one or more household duties, such as helping with homework, taking care of pets, or cooking meals on certain days of the week. By doing so, you will not only be alleviating your significant other's burden but will also take an active role in the lives of your family members.

One of the more challenging things for surgeons (and any medical professional for the matter) to do is to completely disconnect from the workday after they have come home. Your job demands that you stay connected with patients and colleagues given the stakes involved (people's lives), and your partner understands there is never going to be a way that you can 100% disconnect for vast periods of time during the work week. That said, during the work week, it is imperative that when you get home that you carve out some time for your significant other. There is nothing more frustrating for your partner than not getting to fully interact with you even when you are at home because you are mentally still at work. There should be time each day where you truly connect with your partner on something that is important to the two of you. It could be as simple as preparing and eating dinner together, watching your favorite TV show together, or just chatting about each other's days. If you are unable to get out of work mode, talk to your partner, tell them what has you stuck, and have a dialogue with them instead of remaining in work mode. If necessary, put the pager, phone, and laptop in another room so that you don't get tempted to jump back into work. These small connections each day are what will bridge you to the longer periods of time (like vacation) you can spend together where you are unencumbered by the demands of your jobs. Also, not all time is created equal. It goes without saying "quality time" is just that. This means doing activities rather than passively sitting next to one another reading aren't the same—although, obviously there is a time and place for both scenarios.

One of the ways you can maximize the amount of time you can spend together during a normal work week is to look at calendars in advance. Ensure your partner understands the hours of your schedule and looks down the road to find pockets of time that exist where the two of you could go out to a nice dinner, take in a movie, or just veg out together at home if you so choose. The important thing is that by doing this, you are showing your partner how much you value them and how you have the desire to maximize what little time you do have together.

Although managing your schedule to find pockets of time together is nice, it is critical for you and your partner (and if you have one, family) to take longer stretches of time away from your jobs to reconnect as a family. The wear of work (especially a job as taxing as surgeon) can take its toll on any relationship, so make sure you take advantage of all the vacation time that you are allotted per your agreement with your hospital. These longer stretches of time away from work are the times where you both can step back and remember why you chose to be in a relationship and appreciate each other for your non-work qualities. These are the periods of time where you should both be able to recharge your batteries enough to get you to the next period you have together. Vacations don't always have to be lavish either; simple long weekends away to the shore or day trips to an amusement park can remind both of you why you value each other so much.

Finally, when on vacation, it is essential that you leave your work at the hospital. Your partner knows that you care about your patients, but when you are with your partner, you should be with them 100%. There is nothing worse than being in some exotic locale, ready to spend time with the person you care about, only to have them on the phone talking shop. Ensure success on vacation by having a transition plan with some of your colleagues and if necessary your patients. Make sure you have a good plan in place for who is responsible for any issues that come up in the event you are out of the hospital, and make sure your colleagues and patients understand that plan. Creating healthy boundaries like this will prevent every waking minute of your life from being sucked into work and will make for a very happy partner.

One last bit of advice for managing your relationship with your partner is to stay in contact with them during the day, even if it is something as simple as a text to see how they are doing. Staying connected during the day is a great way to see what mood your partner might be in and if some of the daily burdens discussed previously in this chapter might be wearing on them. Keeping the lines of communication open during the day is also a great way for your partner to see how things are going for you during the day and if they need to be a more supportive/encouraging partner if you had a particularly bad day at the office. Collecting these little bits of information during the day allows both of you time to process what is going on in the other's life and adjust accordingly so that you can be the best partner that you can be on that day, whatever might be required of you.

Index

A

ABSITE scores, 20
Academic medicine
  academic positions, 102
  clinical/adjunct instructor, 101
  definition, 101
  surgeon scientist, 102
Academic positions, 102
Accessory dwelling units (ADUs), 120–121
Accountable Care Organization (ACO), 120
Accountant, 139
Accreditation Council for Graduate Medical
  Education (ACGME), 37
Active Duty Tour (ADT), 252
Acute care surgery (ACS), 12, 15, 289
Administrative time, 103
Adult day care, 120
Advice, 130
Affordable Care Act (ACA), 119
Aftercare, 175–177
Air Force and Army and Ensign in the Navy,
  251
American Association for the Surgery of
  Trauma (AAST), 12, 13
American Board of Surgery (ABS), 239, 240
American Burn Association (ABA), 26
American College of Osteopathic Surgeons
  (ACOS) requirements, 242
American College of Surgeons (ACS), 46,
  241, 242, 289
American Society of Bariatric and Metabolic
  Surgeons (ASMBS), 46
American Society of Breast Surgeons
  (ASBrS), 20
American Society of Colon and Rectal
  Surgeons (ASCRS), 31

American Society of Transplant Surgeons
  (ASTS), 56
Anal cancer, 30
Appointments, 157
Assistant professor, 102
Association for Academic Surgeons (AAS),
  289
Association of American Medical Colleges
  (AAMC) report, 83
Attending surgeons
  assessing resident's ability, 182
  relationship between resident and, 183
  resident participation, 182
  teaching basic skills, 182
Attorney, 138, 139, 146–148
Avoiding disasters in operating room
  aftercare, 175
  postoperative checklist, 176
  preparedness
    instrument availability, 174
    patient safety, 172
    physical examination of the surgical
     part, 173
    pre-op note, 172
    preoperative assessment, 173
    reviewing the procedure, 173, 174
    specialists role, 174
  team dynamics, 174

B

Bar code medication administration (BCMA),
  164
Big data, 210
Billing, 140, 154, 155
Blue Cross, 118

Board examination
  ABS, 239
  CE, 240
  oral exam, 240
Bonus, 77, 106, 107, 188
Bookwalter Retractor, 208
Breast Education Self-Assessment Program
  (BESAP), 21
Breast surgical oncology fellowship
  application process, 19–20
  breast conference, 23
  community outreach programs, 23
  educational objectives, 21
  lifestyle, 23–24
  match statistics, 20
  requirements, 22
  schedule, 21
  training program, 22
Bribes, 123
Building a program
  benefits, 141
  leadership role, 142
  patience, time and effort, 143
  planning, 141–142
Burn surgery fellowship
  ABA verification guidelines, 26
  application process, 25
  critical care, 25, 26
  laser therapy, 26
  lifestyle, 26–27
  plastic surgery, 26
  reconstructive surgery, 26
  specialized wound care, 26
Burnout, 191, 192, 279
  spiritual exhaustion, 279
  stress, 280
  withdrawn, 280
Business cards, 200
Business partners, 115–116
Business staff, 137

C
Case selection
  avoiding specific procedure, 196
  elective cases, 197
  emergency call, 197
  procedure list, 196
  surgical approach, 197
Cash-pay business model, 119
Centers for Medicare and Medicaid Services
  (CMS), 120
Central Application Service (CAS), 50

Certifying examination (CE), 240
Changing practices, 258–261
  call referring doctor, 258
  exit strategy, 258
  Medicare inpatient consults *vs.* private
    insurer consults, 259
  planning, 261, 262
  pleasant, 257
  private practice, 258
  procedure codes, 259
  SuperCoder/ACSCodingToday, 260
  switch jobs, 257
  transparency, 259
Chart preparation, 159
Chart, documentation, 145–147
Chief residents, 171
Child labor laws, 189
Chronic stress, 280
Claims-made insurance, 78, 99
Clinic/office hours
  chart preparation, 159
  communication with staff, 161
  documentation, 160
  office procedures, 160, 161
  scheduling, 158, 159
Clinical staff, 137
Clinical/adjunct instructor, 101
Code of medical ethics, 123
Coercion, 123
Colleague-to-colleague communication, 126
Colon and rectal surgery (CRS) fellowship
  application timeline, 34
  board certification, 31
  broadened practice, 32
  CR surgeon, 29
  endoscopic skills, 30
  ERAS, 33
  evolving fiels, 30
  lifestyle, 31
  mentoring, 32–33
  multidisciplinary care, 31
  networking, 33–34
  research, 33
Colon cancer, 30
Colorectal surgery, 257, 258
Communication, 69, 98
Community exposure, 202
Community hospital, 101, 102
Comparison shop, 93
Compensation, 83, 84, 107
Complex general surgical oncology fellowship
  application, 37
  board certification, 37, 39

collaborative approach, 36
complications, 36
interview trail, 37
job search, 38–39
multidisciplinary conferences, 36
multidisciplinary management, 38
nonsurgical rotations, 38
preoperative decision-making, 38
SSO, 37
Computer and phone system equipment,
        135–136
Computer training, 153, 154
Concierge medicine, 119
Conscientious Employee Protection Act, 189
Consultants, 138–139
Consumer-grade medical devices, 210
Continuing care retirement communities
        (CCRCs), 121
Continuing medical education (CME), 78,
        100, 222
    attend regional or national conferences,
        236
    tracking cases, 237
Contract attorney, 75
Contract negotiation
    add-on schedule, 80
    benefits, 78, 79
    bonus structure, 77–78
    call coverage/schedule, 79
    contract attorney, 75–76
    malpractice insurance, 78
    marketing, 80
    noncompete clause, 79
    OR block time, 79
    salary, 76
    staff members, 79
Contract staff, 187
Co-pays, 139
Cover letters, 68–70
Coworkers, 107, 175
Crohn's disease, 30
Cross-country moves, 93
Culture, 190
Curriculum vitae (CV), 67–70
Customer service, 202–203

D
da Vinci surgical system, 247–249
Debt, 132, 137, 140, 251, 261
Demand curve, 118–121
Department of Labor, 188
Depositions, 147–149

Diet, 282
    bad eating habits, 281
    eat low fat, 281
    Meal prep, 282
Digital physician lounges, 289
Digital technologies, 209, 210
Divorce, 298
    costs money, 297
    time, 297–298
    stress, 298
Do not resuscitate (DNR), 170
Doc Halo, 98
Documentation
    EMR, 160
    importance of, 98
    in chart, 145, 146
Donations, 94

E
Early Specialization Program (ESP), 41
Eastern Association for the Surgery of Trauma
        (EAST), 13
Elective surgery, 180
Electronic health records (EHRs), 115, 279
    complications, 168
    feeding information, 165
    IT department, 166
    principles and methods, 165
    system enhancement, 166, 167
Electronic medical records (EMRs), 98
    data exchange, 167
    definition, 163
    history, 164
    note, 126
    system configuration, 166, 167
Electronic personal health records, 163
Electronic Residency Application Service
        (ERAS), 42
Emergency case, 169, 170
Emergency general surgery, see Acute care
        surgery (ACS)
Emergency general surgery (EGS) call, 106
Emergency medical services (EMS), 290
Emotions, 175
Employee break areas, 134
Employee office space, 134
Employment opportunities, 67
Enhanced recovery after surgery (ERAS), 33
Equal Pay Act, 83
Errors, 145, 146
Essential items, 94
Evaluation/management (E&M) codes, 126

Exam rooms, 134
Exam table covering, 136
Experts, 147
Extravagant gift, 124

F
Fair Employment Law, 192
Fair Labor Standards Act, 188
Family planning, 284, 285
Fee-for-service (FFS) model, 118, 120
Fellow of American College of Osteopathic
  Surgeons (FACOS), 241
Fellow of the American College of Surgeons
  (FACS), 241
Fellowship applications
  choosing a residency program, 6
  documents, 3–4
  interviews, 5–6
  mentoring, 4
  networking, 5
  process, 7
  recommendation letters, 5
Fellowship interview
  application review, 8–10
  impressions, 8
  preparation, 9
  respect and deference, 8
Fight, between staff members, 192
Financial advisor, 92
Financial Assistance Program (FAP), 252
Financial planner, 139
Firing staff, 193
First day in clinic, 157, 158
  questions to ask
    appointments, 157
    equipment/supplies, 158
    patient flow, 158
  staffing, 158
First day on job
  credentials submission, 153
  EHR systems, 154
  good impressions, 154
  medical billing, 154, 155
  meeting staffs and physicians, 154
  packing healthy food, 155
  paperwork, 153
  preparing for operation room, 155
  relaxation, 155
  shoes, 155
First emergency case
  anesthesia and operating room staff, 170
  first call, 170

  informed consent, 170
  labs and imaging reports review, 170
  operating room's emergency, 170
  patient history, 169
  seeking help, 170
  staying calm, 169
  time management, 169
First female physician, 82
First job, 107, 108
5-year plan, 255, 256
Free Open Access Medical education
  (FOAM), 289
Full professor, 102
Fundamentals of endoscopic skills, 30
Furniture and fixtures, 133

G
Gender inequality
  knowledge, 84
  professional development, 84
  salary, 84
Gender stereotypes, 82
General office policies, 140
General surgery qualifying examination, 239
General surgery residency programs, 247
Gifts, 123–124
Goals, 141–143
Good impressions, 154
Google health, 163
Graduate Medical Education (GME)
  departments, 92
Guidance, 129
Guide, 129

H
Happiness, 70
Harassment, 192
Having a baby, time to, 283–285
Headhunters, 64
Health Level Seven International (HL7), 167
Health Professions Scholarship Program
  (HPSP), 251, 252
Healthcare dollars, 118, 119
Healthcare economist, 117
Healthcare technology
  consumer-grade medical devices, 210
  digital technologies, 210
  genomics, 210, 211
  medical device, 209
  personalized medicine, 210, 211
  pharmaceuticals, 210, 211

Help, seeking, 129
    assistance during surgery, 179
    difficult case, 180
    elective surgery, 180
    qualified surgeon, 179
    senior opinion, 180
Health Insurance Portability and
        Accountability Act (HIPAA), 224,
        237, 260, 296
Hiring, moving company, 92, 95
Home care, 120
Homeless shelters, 94
Honesty, 145–147
Hospital employment
    happy environment, 107
    hospital support, 107
    salary and bonus, 106
    shifts, 106
    working environment, 107
Hospital privileges, 88
Hospital support, 107

I

Identification and credentials, 95
Incentive, 188
Independent model, 49
Inflammatory bowel disease (IBD), 30
Information technology (IT) department, 166
Informed consent, 170
Innovation
    commercialization of intellectual property,
        207
    compensation, 208
    product development and improvement, 208
    production, 208
    protection of intellectual property, 207
    sales and marketing, 208
Insurance, 99, 118–120
Insurance companies, 138
Insurance enrollment, 88
Insurance panels, 154
Integrated model, 49
Integrated vascular surgery track, 41
Intellectual property
    commercialization, 207
    protection of, 207
Interacting with residents
    autonomy, 214
    confidence, 219
    education, 215
    honesty, 219
    human, 219

knowledgeable, 219
    listens, 219
    personas to avoid
        best friend, 216
        guilt tripper, 217
        my way, 218
        over sharer, 216
        town gossip, 217
    present, 219
    respect, 213, 214, 219
    setting high standards, 220
    successful mentor, 218
    supportive, 219
    team player, 219
Internet is forever, 288–290
Internet/websites, 164
Interview day, 72
Interview process, 5–6, 71, 72
    first impression, 71
    follow-up, 73
    interview day, 72
    plastic surgery fellowship, 50–51
    preparation
        faculty and future partners, 72
        research on institution, 71
        travel plan, 72
    transplant fellowship, 57
Intimate gift, 124
Intraoperative picture, 126, 127

J

Job application
    application submission, 69
    communication with current program, 69
    cover letters, 68
    CVs, 68
    multiple interviews, 69
    preparation, 67
    resume, 68
    salary, 70
    term sheet, 69
Job safety, 189
Job search
    academic positions, 63, 64
    geographical location, 63
    headhunters, 64
    location, 105
    locum companies, 64, 65
    private practices, 64
    specialty website, 64
    word of mouth, 65
Jurisprudence exam, 87

K
KevinMD, 289
Kitchenware, 94

L
Laparoscopic surgery, 249
Lawsuits, 98, 99
  depositions, 147
  experts, 147
  malpractice cases, 145
Lawyer, 146, 147
Leadership development, 263
  authority, 265
  consensus, 265
  ideas and power in numbers, 264
  overlap of purpose, 264
  physical force, 263
  power poses and influence in presence,
    265, 266
  reciprocity, 265
  scarcity, 265
  social norms, 264
  state action, 264
  wealth, 264
Leadership role, 142–143
Learning new procedure
  collect own data and stay with literature,
    246
  MIS, 245
  preceptor preparation, 246
  sleeve gastrectomy, 245, 246
Leaving first job, 108
Legal document, 145
Legal fees, 76
Licensure, 78, 87–88
Loan, 78

M
Maintenance of Certification (MOC)
  components of, 235, 236
  grand rounds, morbidity and mortality
    conference, 236
  tracking cases, 237, 238
Maintenance staff, 137
Malpractice
  communication, 98
  coverage, 99
  documentation, 98
  quality of care, 98
  rules for physician, 99–100
Malpractice cases, 145–147

Malpractice insurance, 78
Marketing, 80, 125–127
Maternity/paternity leave, 79
Medical billing, 154, 155
Medical economics
  ACA, 119
  ACO, 120
  demand curve, 119
  FFS model, 120
  healthcare economists, 117
  supply and demand, 118
Medical errors, 97, 100
Medical Group Management Association
    (MGMA), 76, 77
Medical practice
  assisting surgeons, 201
  breakfast/lunch with physicians, 200, 201
  community exposure, 202
  customer service, 202
  professional exposure, 201, 202
  taking calls, 201
  visiting referrals, 200
Medical record, 98
Medical supplies, 136
Medical/surgical supply procurement advisory
    services, 136
Medicare, 88, 120, 181, 223, 259, 260
Medscape Physician Compensation Report, 83
Mentorship, 129, 130
Microblogs, 290
Microsoft HealthVault, 163
Military surgery
  ADTs, 252
  benefits, 252
  deployments, 253
  FAP, 252
  fellowships, 252
  HPSP program, 252
  scholarship, 251
Mindfulness, 291–293
  among the residents, 294, 295
  around the hospital, 294
  at home, 296
  Don't Sweat the Small Stuff, 291
  patient care, 295
  trauma, 293
Minimally invasive surgery fellowship (MIS),
    245
  application process, 45–46
  applications fees, 46
  ASMBS, 47
  components, 47
  Fellowship Council, 45, 47

practicing option, 47
  resources, 48
Mistakes, 145, 146
Mobile apps, 164
Moving
  costs, 92
  downsizing, 93–94
  family and friends, 92
  personal movers, 92–93
  professional movers, 93
  scheduling, 91
  survival kit, 94
Moving truck rentals, 93
Multiple interviews, 69

N

National Accreditation Program for Breast
      Centers (NAPBC), 23
National Labor Relations Act of 1935, 188
National Resident Matching Program (NRMP)
      system, 3, 15, 34, 56
National Women Physician day, 82
New England Journal of Medicine, 97
New job as surgeon, 155
Noncompete clause, 79
Nonverbal communication, 98

O

Occupational Safety and Health Act, 188
Occurrence insurance, 78, 99
Office hours, 157–161
Office of the National Coordinator for
      Healthcare Technology (ONC), 163
Office policies, 139–140
Office procedures, 160, 161
On-site first interview, 69
Operating room facilities, 134, 135
OR block time, 79
OR coverage, 106
Organ Procurement and Transplantation
      Network (OPTN), 57
Orientation process, 153, 154

P

Paperwork, 87–89, 95, 153
Partners
  business, 115
  personal, 116
Patient death, communication, 206
Patient gowns, 136

Patient safety, 171, 172, 180
Patient waiting room, 133
Performance improvement plan (PIP), 193
Personal health records (PHRs), 163, 164
Personal introduction, 200
Personal movers, 92, 93
Personal partners, 116
Personnel decisions, 137
Phone calls, 125, 126
Phone interview, 69
Phone operator, 138
Physical office space, 131–133
Physician information profile, 50
Physician transparency, 210
Plastic surgery, 26
Plastic surgery fellowship
  application process, 50–51
  expense, 51–52
  independent model, 49
  integrated model, 49
  integrated/independent programs, 52
  interviews, 51
  match, 52
  preparation, 52
  research, 53
  resources, 53
  subspecialty, 53
Postoperative checklist, 176
Practicing, in academic setting, 104
Prejudice, 84
Pre-op note, 172, 173
Preparedness, 172–174
Private practice, 105, 106, 258
Privileges, 88
Productivity bonus, 106, 107
Professional attire, 72
Professional exposure, 201, 202
Professional movers, 93
Professional online presence, *see* Social media
Professionalism, 72, 221, 222, 224, 290
  accountability, 222, 223
  appearance, 225
  charter, 221
  expertise, 222
  Hippocratic Oath, 221
  honesty/integrity/confidentiality/ethics,
      224
  respect for yourself and others, 223
  responsibility, 222, 223
  timeliness, 223, 224
Program directors, 67–69
Programs of All-Inclusive Care for the Elderly
      (PACE), 121

Q
Quality of care, 98
Quality picture, 126, 127

R
Receptionist, 138
Recruiters, 68, 69
Recruiting firms, 186
Rectal cancer, 30
Recycling centers, 94
Referrals, 126, 185, 191
Referring physicians, 125–127
Refugee centers, 94
Registered Physician in Vascular Interpretation
  (RPVI) certification, 43
Reimbursement, 92
Relocation, 91, 92
Relocation reimbursement, 78
Rescue surgery, 12–13
Research, 227, 232, 233
  clinical volume, 229
  closing, 233
  communication with mentors and
    collaborator, 229
  coordination, 230
  meeting, 229
  mentoring, 231–232
  negotiation and contracts, 228, 229
  space, 230
  support
    financial, 232
    grant submissions, 232
    personal, 233
  teamwork, 230
  vision, 227, 228
  write, 231
Residents in operating room
  abilities, 181, 182
  participation, 182
  patient safety, 181
  procedure list, 196
  relationship between attending surgeons
    and, 183
Resource identification, 103
Respite care, 121
Rest, surgeon, 99
Resumes, 68
Retention bonus, 77
Revenue, 106, 107
Right staff
  candidate diligence, 186

interview, 186
negotiating salary, 186
recruiting firms, 186
referral, 185
training, 189, 190
website, 185
Risk management office, 148
Risk management officer, 146
Robotic surgery, 249
  advanced minimally invasive fellowships,
    247
  barriers, 248–249
  colorectal surgery, 249
  general surgery residency programs, 247
  revision surgery, 249
  robotic hernia, 249
  3D visualization and wristed instruments,
    249
  training, 247, 248
Romance, in workplace, 192

S
Salary, 70, 76–77, 107, 188
San Francisco Match (SF Match), 50
Scheduling patients, 196
Scientific Registry of Transplant Recipients
  (SRTR), 57
Selling, 93, 94
Setting up office
  consultants, 138
  electronic medical records, 135
  employee break areas, 134
  employee office space, 134
  exam rooms, 134
  furniture and fixtures, 133
  IT and telephone systems, 135
  medical supplies, 136
  office policy, 139
  operating room, 134, 135
  patient waiting room, 133
  personnel decision
    answering service, 138
    business staff, 137
    clinical staff, 137
    insurance companies, 138
    phone operator, 138
    receptionist, 138
  physical office space
    ADA, 133
    location, 132
    ordinance requirements, 132

parking space, 132
  rent/own, 132
  sign, 132
  private office space, 133
  website, 135, 136
Sexual harassment, 192
Shifts, 106
Sign-on bonus, 77
Sleeve gastrectomies, 245, 246
Social media, 287
  blogs and microblogs, 289, 290
  internet is forever, 288, 290
  online rating, 288, 289
  physician communities, 289
Socialized medicine, 119
Society of American Gastrointestinal
  and Endoscopic Surgeons
  (SAGES), 46
Society of Surgical Oncology (SSO), 19, 37
Spouse, 116
SSO Online Match System Application, 19
Stabilization Act of 1942, 118
Staff
  burnout, 191
  contract staff, 187
  culture, 190
  employment laws, 188, 189
  firing, 193
  performance, 190–191
  salary, 188
  temporary staff, 187
  training, 189, 190
  using resource effectively, 187
  workplace challenges, 192
Strategic planning, 142
Stress management, 175, 276
  medical education, 276, 277
  mitigation strategies, 276
  physician development, 275
  problem-solving economy, 277
  remediation and practice, 277
  stress, definition, 275
Structured repayment plans, 140
Student loan repayment, 78
Successful practice, 131, 134
Successful team, 143
Sue, 145, 148
Supply and demand, 118–119
Supply curve, 120
Surgeon partner empathy, 300
Surgeon personal relationship management, 302
Surgeon scientist, 102–104

Surgeon Specific Registry (SSR), 237
Surgeon spouse perspective, 299–302
Surgeon time management, 302
Surgery homework, 160
Surgical Council on Resident Education
  (SCORE), 39
Surgical Critical Care and Acute Care Surgery
  Fellowship Application Service
  (SAFAS), 13
Surgical critical care fellowship, 105, 106
  amount of applicants and fellowship spots,
    15
  application, 13, 14
  board certification, 11
  critically ill trauma, 11
  fellowship years, 16
  interview process, 14, 15
  match day, 15
  program selection, 13
  surgical patients, 11
Surgical emergency, 170
Surgical ICU, 106
Surgical oncology, 125
Survival kit, 94–95

T
Tail coverage, 78, 99
Teaching responsibilities, 181–183
Teaching surgeon, 171
Team dynamics, 174–175
Team work, 142, 143
Temporary staff, 187
10-year plan, 256
Term sheet, 69
Throwing away, 93, 94
Thyroidectomy, 292
TigerText, 98
Tools, 95
Towels and toiletries, 94
Traditional vascular fellowship track, 41
Training staff, 189, 190
Transplant fellowship
  applications, 56
  ASTS website, 56
  interview, 57–59
  OPTN, 57
  personal statements, 56
  ranking, 57–60
  recommendation letter, 56
  resources, 60
  SRTR, 57

Trauma, 293
    care, 105, 106
    critical care fellowship, 11, 12
    surgeons, 106, 107
Travel costs, 92
Travel plan, 72
Typed message, 126

U
Ulcerative colitis, 30
Unfamiliar instrumentation, 174
US Drug Enforcement Administration
        (DEA), 88

V
Vascular Interpretation (PVI) exam, 43
Vascular surgery certifying exam, 43
Vascular surgery fellowship
    application process, 41–42
    boards, 43
    job opportunities, 44
    quality of life, 42
    quality of training, 41–43

    research, 43
    resources, 44
    vascular lab, 43
Vascular Surgery Qualifying Exam, 43

W
Wage discrimination, 83
Website, 185
Women
    in history, 82
    salary, 84
    wage discrimination, 83
Work challenges, 129, 130
Work-life balance, 271–273
Work relative value units (wRVUs), 77
Work-life balance, 129
Workplace issues
    fight between staff members, 192
    harassment, 192
    romance, 192

X
XPRIZE, 209

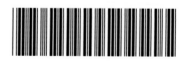